Music as Medicine
particularly in Parkinson's

Daphne Bryan PhD

A self-help book suggesting ways
music can help health problems.

No knowledge of music is needed
to use the ideas in this book.

**Clink
Street**

London | New York

Published by Clink Street Publishing 2020

Copyright © 2020

First edition.
The author asserts the moral right under the Copyright, Designs and Patents Act 1988 to be identified as the author of this work.

ISBNs:
978-1-913340-58-2 paperback
978-1-913340-59-9 ebook

I would like to dedicate this book to all the new friends with Parkinson's who I have met, whether face to face, by telephone, Skype or email, since my diagnosis. Thank you all for your help, encouragement, support and friendship.

Contents

Chapter 4: Making music   **35**

Chapter 5: On a personal note...   **57**

Appendices   **65**

References   **75**

About the Author

Daphne Bryan began playing the piano at the age of seven and at 13 was awarded a county scholarship to study piano and voice. She continued her studies at music college, where she was awarded the piano prize in her second year.

After college, Daphne taught music in schools in Salford, London and Hampshire and then in British Forces schools in Germany and Belgium. During this time, she also taught piano privately and trained several choirs.

At the age of 51, she gained an MA with distinction from Sheffield University in Psychology for Musicians and, four years later, a PhD in music psychology.

In 2010, she was diagnosed with Parkinson's. Since then she has researched keenly to find ways in which she can positively influence her health. Music has provided many ways through which she has reduced her symptoms.

She still teaches piano and trains a choir.

Foreword

An informed, clear and easy to follow introduction to the new science of music medicine and its possible applications to the treatment of neurological disorders.

Dr Joaquin Farias
Director of the Neuroplastic Training Institute in Toronto
A leading specialist treating dystonia and movement disorders.

Chapter 1

Introduction

*"Music can heal wounds
which medicine cannot touch."*

DEBASISH MRIDHA

Music is an important component of many of our lives, whether we prefer rock or reggae, hymn or hip hop, Glastonbury or Glyndebourne. In fact, it would be hard to live a life without hearing music as it is used in shops and restaurants, accompanies films and advertisements and often provides background sound in the workplace. Yet how many of us are aware of how music affects our body, brain and mood?

This book is the result of my personal search for ways in which I, as a person with Parkinson's, could use music to improve my quality of life. I based my search on relevant published studies where, I felt, ideas had been tested on many participants. The studies will only be reported briefly, but anyone who is interested in more detail can find the articles mentioned in the references at the back of the book. Author and year will be given in brackets in the chapter. Although there will be particular focus on Parkinson's Disease, many of the symptoms discussed are experienced by people with other diagnoses and by people who are otherwise fit and healthy. I also wanted to write this as a self-help book as opportunities to work with music therapists are rare for most people with Parkinson's, and furthermore, I wanted to make sure that the practical suggestions I gave could be implemented to improve symptoms whether the person thought themselves musical or not.

What is Parkinson's Disease?

Parkinson's Disease is a complex chronic neurological condition which affects predominantly dopamine-producing neurons in a specific part of the brain called the substantia nigra. As a consequence of this, a range of bodily functions become affected. Although Parkinson's is characterised mainly by slowly worsening movement problems such as resting tremor, rigidity and bradykinesia (slowness of movement), there are many other symptoms people with Parkinson's report: sleep disturbance, anxiety, depression, apathy, voice and swallowing problems, loss of a sense of smell, cognitive impairment, constipation, gait disturbance and freezing to highlight only a few. Symptoms only become noticeable when a significant amount of neurons have been lost or damaged which can be ten or fifteen years into the condition.

Parkinson's UK estimates that 145,000 people were diagnosed with Parkinson's in the UK in 2018, and allowing for population growth and ageing, propose that this is likely to increase to around 168,000 people by 2025. They also suggest that one in 37 people alive today will be diagnosed with Parkinson's at some point in their life. In the U.S., the Parkinson's Foundation estimates that nearly one million will be living with Parkinson's in the U.S. by 2020, with approximately 60,000 Americans being diagnosed each year. Their estimate of the worldwide figure for people with Parkinson's is around ten million.

The cause of Parkinson's remains largely unknown. Although current medication helps symptoms, it does not slow or halt disease progression. Furthermore, current pharmacotherapy is associated with unwanted side effects, such as dyskinesia, dystonia, motor fluctuations, oedema, somnolence, dizziness, and hallucinations (Stowe et al 2008). Most people with Parkinson's will die with it rather than of it, and if a person is diagnosed in their 60s, for example, they can live for many years with the condition. As the standard medication does not address all the many symptoms and can often cause unwanted side-effects, any complementary therapy that can improve quality of life needs to be recognised and utilised. This book aims to show how music may offer safe, self-help approaches which might help to reduce various symptoms.

Music used for healing throughout history

Using music to heal body and affect mood is not new. In the course of human history, music has been used not only as an art form but also as a tool for healing. Frescoes dating from 4000 BC, depicting harp playing priests and musicians, are probably the oldest examples which suggest that music was believed to have healing properties at that time.

In the Bible's Old Testament, Saul was said to suffer from depressive symptoms and his servants suggested that they find someone who was a "cunning player on the harp" (1 Samuel chapter 16 v 16 Revised Version).

"And it came to pass, when the evil spirit from God was upon Saul, that David took the harp, and played with his hand: so Saul was refreshed, and was well, and the evil spirit departed from him." (1 Samuel Chapter 16 v 23. Revised Version)

The ancient Greeks developed music as therapy, with Pythagoras proposing that body and soul could be influenced by music, through the understanding of music's law and order (Dobrzinska et al 2006). The Pythagoreans employed music in their daily routine, playing music before bedtime to calm them and provide a good night's sleep with pleasant dreams. On waking, they would play particular compositions on the lyre to shake off sleep and prepare them for the rigours of the day.

The philosopher Plato considered music to be "the medicine of the soul" (Gfeller 2002). He claimed in *The Republic*:

"Music is most sovereign because rhythm and harmony find their way to the inmost soul and take strongest hold upon it, imparting grace, if one is rightly trained."

Aristotle also believed in music's ability to heal, seeing it as providing relief from negative emotions (Dobrzinska et al 2006). He had a theory that song, wine, and women were the three necessary components to create an optimal environment for man (Ansdell 2004).

Many primitive cultures considered music an important part of everyday life. Native Americans used music in their healing rituals, often in the form of singing and chanting with percussive instruments. The United States Indian Bureau contains 1,500 songs used by Native Americans for healing purposes. In the Middle Ages, the importance of music for keeping well was so highly regarded that the law mandated that those studying medicine should also appreciate music. At this time, specific musical applications were suggested for particular medical problems, for example, music which alternated flute and harp was believed to be a remedy for gout.

A plague occurred in Germany in 1374 in which sufferers danced uncontrollably till they became unconscious through exhaustion. Thousands died, and more outbreaks occurred across Europe over the next two centuries. The only way of stopping the mania was to have a musician play for the afflicted dancer (Harvey 1980). At a similar time, the illness tarantism, thought to be caused by the bite of a tarantula, was believed to be cured by listening and dancing to the music of a 'tarantella', a folk dance with a fast, upbeat tempo. It is possible that the wild dancing helped the problem by separating the venom from the sufferer's blood.

During the Renaissance, music continued to be used to treat mania and depression. The Italian sixteenth century theorist, Gioseffo Zarlino, believed that musical harmony had healing abilities. He suggested music could be used to relieve pain, depression, mania, the plague and even restore hearing. In 1899, an article in *The Lancet* by J.T.R. Davison titled 'Music in Medicine' led to the now growing interest in investigating music and health (Davison 1899).

For many thousands of years, therefore, people have believed music to have a place in healing, but what properties in music give it this power?

Why is music so special?

Recent advances in neuroscience, brain imaging and technology have made it possible to study exactly what response happens in the brain when a person listens to music. Finnish researchers, using functional magnetic resonance imaging (fMRI) discovered that music does something to the brain that no other stimulus does: it lights up more of the brain than any other activity (Alluri et al 2011). The researchers recorded the brain responses of individuals who were listening to a piece of modern Argentinian tango and were able to analyse which features of the music, pulse, rhythm, tone, timbre etc. caused which part of the brain to be activated. They discovered that listening to music stimulates more than just the auditory areas of the brain: that processing musical pulse used motor areas in the brain, that limbic areas of the brain were involved with rhythm and tonality processing, and that the so-called default mode network, assumed to be associated with mind-wandering and creativity, was used to process timbre.

The fact that music stimulates so much of the brain is the key to its usefulness in treating neurological conditions, because it can activate parts of the brain that are working normally which are then able to compensate for areas which are damaged. An amazing demonstration of this can be seen when a person with Parkinson's becomes frozen, unable to lift their feet and move forward, but when music is played it is as though a switch has been flicked in the brain and they are able to walk forward easily and with confidence. This will be discussed in Chapter 3 'Moving to music'.

Music is special, too, because of 'entrainment', where internal physiological rhythms, such as brain waves, pulse and blood pressure synchronise with the music. How this can be used to reduce Parkinson's symptoms will be discussed in Chapter 2 'Listening to music', while Chapter 4, 'Making music' will explore the very important benefits of singing and playing a musical instrument.

Although this book focuses on the symptoms associated with Parkinson's, many of these may be experienced by the wider population and, therefore, this book could be of use to all.

Chapter 2

Listening to music

"My heart, which is so full to overflowing, has often been solaced and refreshed by music when sick and weary."

MARTIN LUTHER

The aim of this chapter is to explore the benefits of simply listening to music. Most of us spend time every day listening in various situations: at home on the radio or a CD, through earphones as we exercise, on a car audio system, or at a concert. According to a report released by Nielson Music in 2017 (www.marketingcharts.com), the average American spends more than four and a half hours a day listening to music, while a UK survey found that most respondents spent up to two hours, with 5% spending as many as seven hours or more listening per day. (www.statista.com/statistics). Most of us listen to music, therefore, but are we aware of the effect which it has on our brains, bodies and mood?

This chapter will look at the symptoms – anxiety, insomnia, depression, pain and brain fog – experienced by many in the general population as well as with Parkinson's. It will investigate how listening to music can offer help with these symptoms as well as advising on the types of music and the particular characteristics it needs to have to be beneficial.

Anxiety

Anxiety can be described as a feeling of uneasiness and worry, usually generalised and unfocussed, which is often an overreaction to a situation that is only subjectively seen as menacing. Up to 40% of Parkinson's patients experience clinically significant anxiety (Walsh & Bennett 2001). Current thinking suggests that anxiety may not only be a psychological reaction to the stress of the disease but may also be a product of the neurological changes of the condition itself. Often anxiety and depression precede the motor symptoms that lead to diagnosis. A study, collecting information from clinical interviews, found that patients often experienced anxiety and/or depression up to 25 years before their motor symptoms were identified (Seritan et al 2019).

Anxiety is not only a symptom which reduces quality of life in itself but which can also cause a significant worsening of other disease symptoms (Routh 1987). Pimenta et al (2018) found that anxiety contributed to a greater freezing of gait. Unsurprisingly, just as people without Parkinson's often shake when anxious, it can also make a Parkinson's tremor worse. Therefore, any safe approach to reduce anxiety will also help other symptoms and the condition generally.

There appears to be little or no research that has looked into the effect of relaxing music on anxiety in Parkinson's specifically, but there are many studies that have considered the effect of music on anxiety in other medical situations.

The first published experiment using music to relax patients was conducted as early as 1914, and describes the effects of using the phonograph, an early form of gramophone, in operating and recovery rooms to reduce the need for pharmacological analgesia and reduce anxiety in patients undergoing the 'horrors of surgery' (Kane 1914).

More recent studies have found that listening to relaxing music while awaiting surgery reduced anxiety in patients to a greater extent and with fewer side effects than medication (Bringman et al 2009). Voss et al (2004) found that patients recovering from open-heart surgery found listening to music was more effective at relaxing them than scheduled rest and treatment. A Chinese study in the *Journal of Clinical Nursing* found that for patients on mechanical ventilation, listening to music proved a simple and safe nursing intervention to allay anxiety (Lee et al 2005), while a feasibility study, looking at music intervention for 150 critically ill patients, reported their anxiety had reduced after music sessions (Fallek et al 2019). So what is happening physiologically when we listen to relaxing music?

Scientists have discovered that music can promote what is referred to as 'entrainment', the body's ability to synchronise its internal rhythms with the external rhythms of the music being listened to, and several studies have set out to measure various physiological effects of listening to music.

Bradt et al (2013) found that when coronary heart disease patients listened to music it reduced their heart rate, respiratory rate and blood pressure and Watchi et al (2007) notes that the relaxing properties of music – in this case some slow movements from Mozart's piano sonatas – can reduce inflammatory markers and strengthen the immune system.

Relaxing music has also been seen to affect cortisol levels. Cortisol is a hormone, and among other things, it is produced by the body to help it respond to stress. Cortisol levels were monitored in a study where the participants were undergoing an operation with spinal anaesthesia and light sedation. The patients, who were therefore awake, were either played orchestral music or 'a pleasant auditory stimulus' (non-musical), to reduce theatre noise. The researchers found that the individuals who listened to music during the operation had lower cortisol levels and required less anaesthetic (Koelsch et al 2011). Khalfa et al (2003) measured the cortisol levels of students recovering after a period of stress and found that the levels of those who listened to relaxing music decreased far quicker than those of the control group who followed their period of stress with a time of silence.

Even babies, it appears, have the mental capacity to be entrained. When a study compared singing to calm a baby rather than talking to the baby it was found that singing to babies calmed them for up to twice as long as being talked to (Peretz et al 2015).

As we have seen, there is considerable research showing that listening to relaxing music can reduce anxiety in quite stressful situations. This is not only 'felt' by people but has been measurable in physiological changes such as reduced pulse rate, normalised blood pressure, decreased cortisol levels etc. But what type of music is relaxing?

Music has various components; beat, tempo, rhythm, melody, harmony, texture, form, etc. To relax us, music needs to have a slow tempo. If we think of our body entraining to the music, the pulse of the music needs to be similar to a relaxed pulse – between 60 and 70 beats per minute. Gentle melodies with slow stable rhythms on instruments such as flute, guitar or piano are conducive to relaxation. Many styles of music have examples which fit these basic prerequisites, including:

- Classical
- Light jazz
- Easy listening
- Classical Indian music using voice and/or veena
- Native American music

I have included a range of examples in 'Appendix 1' at the back of the book and suggest you listen on YouTube, Spotify or iTunes etc. and select your own playlist of relaxing music. It is best that you *like* the music you choose. If it irritates you, you will not relax!

So how do you take this musical medicine and what is the dosage? For the biggest effect on anxiety it would be best if you stop what you are doing and sit or lie somewhere warm and comfortable, so that you can fully relax while you absorb the musical sounds. However, if it is not possible to stop to listen, it will have some effect on anxiety if played as background as you go about your day.

While we are discussing relaxing music, we shall look at another symptom which can also be helped by listening to this style of music.

Insomnia

Insomnia is a frequent complaint in patients with Parkinson's (Gjerstad et al 2007), and, like anxiety, it is not only a symptom in itself. The tiredness insomnia causes can make other symptoms worse. Furthermore, insomnia can be aggravated by other Parkinson's symptoms like stiffness and slowness which make turning over in bed or getting comfortable difficult. A tremor can also interfere with getting to or staying asleep. Additionally, some Parkinson's medications can interfere with sleep patterns (Van Hilton et al 1994).

Once again there is a lack of studies looking at the effect of music on insomnia specifically in Parkinson's, but quite a few studies which show the benefits of music for improving sleep amongst other groups. One such study, whose 60 participants, aged between 60 and 83, all of whom reported difficulty in sleeping pre-study, listened to 45-minutes of sedative music tapes at bedtime. This resulted in longer sleep duration, less sleep disturbance and less daytime dysfunction. Furthermore, their sleep improved week on week, suggesting a cumulative effect (Lai & Good 2005). Chang et al (2005) found that 25 chronic insomnia sufferers assigned randomly to a 'music' group had significantly better scores for rested rating, shortened stage 2 sleep and prolonged REM sleep compared to the control group. Also a study which looked at the effect of music on patients in a medical intensive care unit found that those who listened to music had significantly lower heart rates and reported that they felt their sleep quality had improved (Su et al 2013).

Harmat et al (2008) monitored 94 students (aged 19–28) with sleep complaints, dividing them into three groups; one given classical music, one an audiobook and the third group with no intervention. The group who were given the music input, listening for 45-minutes before bed, found that music consistently improved their sleep quality where the other interventions had had no effect. Finally, a meta-analysis of ten randomised studies on the subject of sleep, involving 557 participants, found that sleep quality was improved significantly by listening to music before bedtime (Wang et al 2014).

Researchers think that music has this effect on sleep because it acts upon the central nervous system and has anti-anxiety and relaxing effects. It is also suggested that it may impact on the production of compounds like opioids and oxytocin, which are believed to improve sleep. There is a lot of evidence that suggests that music aids sleep, and because it is easy to use and has no side effects, it is well worth trying.

Most of the studies mentioned above, asked their participants to listen for 45-minutes at bedtime, which seems a reasonable time period to try if you wish to do your own trial. And even if for some of the time the music is used to provide background atmosphere as final preparations are made for bed, I suggest that at least 30 minutes is spent in bed, just relaxing and listening. As one study notes (Wang et al 2014), for chronic sleep disorders, music showed a cumulative dose effect, so try it for at least three weeks.

The music which is suitable for insomnia is the same as the relaxing music recommended for anxiety, so you might like to listen to some of the examples in Appendix 1 and select pieces that you enjoy to create a playlist.

Depression

Depression is a common symptom of Parkinson's. One estimate is that 35% of Parkinson's patients have depression (Aarsland et al 2011), while Parkinson's Foundation estimates that 50% of those diagnosed will experience some form of depression at some time during their illness. Depression is a mood disorder in which a person experiences great feelings of sadness, loss and hopelessness to the extent that it interferes with their ability to function.

There are various possible causes of depression in Parkinson's. A person may experience grief at being diagnosed as they realise that the future they had expected could well be very different. Changes in the brain, particularly in the areas that produce dopamine, norepinephrine and serotonin, which affect mood, energy, motivation and sleep, can lead to depression. Later in the disease, the difficulty living with a chronic disease and the limitations it brings with it can result in depression. One study found the severity and frequency of depression appeared more in early and late stage Parkinson's compared to the middle stage (Starkstein et al 1990).

Once again, there is a lack of research into the effect of listening to music on depression in Parkinson's, though there are many studies which have considered the effect of music on mood in other groups. Two studies looked into the effect of listening to music on depressed older adults, and both showed statistically-significant decreases in depression scores (Chan et al 2009, 2010). The researchers make the point that older people do not always regard depression as a treatable disorder and often find it difficult to express themselves verbally. It was suggested that listening to music allowed people to feel they were expressing their inner feelings without having to put them into words.

Two other studies looked into the effect of listening to music on students with depression (Harmat et al 2008, Esfandiari & Mansouri 2014). Both found that their participants' depressive symptoms decreased significantly after they had listened to music. One of the studies compared the effect of listening to light music to listening to fast, heavy music and found that, in the study, both styles of music decreased depression.

Several studies have considered the effect of listening to sad music in particular, (Garrido & Schibert 2013, Shifriss et al 2014). They found that sad music lowered mood and the participants preferred to listen to happy music if they were feeling low. However, two other studies, which compared the music listening choice (sad or happy) of depressed participants and healthy controls, found that their depressed participants were more likely to choose *sad* music compared to their healthy counterparts (Millgram et al 2015, Yoon et al 2019). The reason the participants gave was that listening to sad music made them happier, which raises the question: how can sad music make a sad person happier?

The most mainstream psychological explanation is to do with social comparison, where the person who listens to the sad music feels better because the musician they are listening to sounds a lot worse! Another explanation is that listening to sad music causes the body to release opiates as the body prepares for the traumatic event, which, as it is only in the music, leaves the listener with a body full of opiates and nothing bad to allay. Also, as mentioned earlier, listening to sad music might be a way of expressing an emotion that the listener feels unable to verbalise themselves, but which, through the music, they are able to get off their chests (Van den Tol et al 2016). Participants with depression in another study said that they chose to listen to sad music because it was low in energy levels and had a calming effect (Yoon et al 2019). But what characteristics make music sad? Obviously if music has lyrics which express a sad emotion then that will help to make a song seem sad, but what in the music itself makes it carry a sad emotion?

Firstly, sad music is usually in a minor key. There are two common modes used in Western music; major mode which sounds bright and happy and minor mode which sounds darker and sadder. The mode is made minor or major by the particular seven note scale used for the composition. Given two pieces with the same keynote, one in the major and one in the minor mode, there is basically just one note which always differs, the 3rd note above the keynote. In the minor mode the 3rd is a half-step lower than it is in the major mode. The 3rd is an important note in a key particularly because it is one of the three notes which form the key chord, the main chord used in the harmony. This small difference between the 3rd note in the minor compared to the 3rd in the major mode colours both melody and harmony and makes a musical composition in a minor key sound darker.

Secondly, the speed of the piece affects the emotion of a piece. Fast-moving pieces generally sound happier than slow music. If speed and tonality are combined, different effects result. For example, fast music in a major key will sound happy but in a minor key will probably sound angry. Add pitch to this and you have other emotions, such as high-pitched music played quietly will sound sinister, but if played loudly will probably sound happy unless it is in a minor key (Gabrielsson & Lindstrom 2010). Melodic shape, too, can carry emotion with it as can harmonies and harmonic progression.

Beyond the characteristics of the music as written, emotion can be affected by a musician's performance. A good musician interprets a composition using subtle variations in tempo, dynamics and phrasing while still staying true to the written composition. This can affect the emotional feel of a piece as noticed when the same composition is performed by different musicians.

Then there is the effect of context and memory. A piece of music can often carry with it memories of the time it was first listened to, so will be affected by what other things were happening at that time. The song 'Sealed with a Kiss' sung in the early 1960s by Brian Hyland will always be particularly sad for me as I listened to it endlessly while suffering my first teenage break-up! Processing music and language, specifically memorising information, uses some of the same brain systems which explains how particular music can bring up clear memories, a tool which has been so important in stimulating early memories for dementia patients. Researchers have also found that music we heard as teenagers may have a greater emotional link to our brain than anything we hear as an adult.

If you wish to listen to some sad music in the hope that, for any of the reasons previously suggested, it might make you feel happier, I have listed some examples in Appendix 2. If they make you feel sad or sadder please stop listening! I have included Barber's 'Adagio for strings', a piece which Thomas Larson has declared 'The Saddest Music Ever Written' in a book of the same name. It has been used at a number of high-profile memorials: Presidents Franklin Roosevelt and John F. Kennedy, Albert Einstein and Grace Kelly. It was also played at a London Promenade concert after 9/11 and I chose it for my father's funeral. At the time, my young daughter, unwittingly recognising the power of connection and memory, commented that we would never be able to listen to the piece again.

In summary, most studies suggest that listening to music can help ease depression. Whether this music should be sad or happy is not clear from studies. Most did find, however, that self-selected music had a more successful outcome. So, if you feel depressed, listen to some suggestions in the appendices and make a playlist. Find somewhere comfortable to relax and see if listening lifts your spirits.

Pain

Parkinson's is most often associated with tremor and rigidity and is less widely seen as a disease which causes a variety of pain syndromes. However, causes of pain in Parkinson's are numerous. These include muscular stiffness, dystonia, dyskinesia, musculoskeletal pain, joint pain, neuropathy, and abdominal pain, to name the most common (Ford 2010). Furthermore, higher perceived pain correlated in one study with depression, demonstrating that if you are depressed you will also feel any pain you have more strongly (Rana 2018).

Researchers have explored the effect of music on various situations where pain is considerable; chronic non-malignant pain which persists in spite of traditional interventions (Siedlieck & Good 2006), pain during rehabilitation after total knee replacement surgery (Hsu et al 2017), pain during labour (Simavli et al 2014), and on fibromyalgia pain (Garza-Villarreal et al 2014). All studies found that listening to music reduced pain and analgesic requirement. One qualitative study explored the narratives of eleven people living with chronic pain. The researchers reported that music could improve emotional state and uplift, console, energise and relax the listener and offer a sense of companionship. It could also act as a distraction from pain, as a cue to movement and as a motivator to exercise. Finally, music could provide a link to memories of a life before pain and a means of escape from a painful body (Gold & Clare 2012). These studies suggest that music has the power to reduce quite wide-ranging pain, and therefore, has something to offer the Parkinson's patient with this problem.

Brain Fog

People with Parkinson's often complain of 'brain fog' or more specifically, problems with concentration, multi-tasking, problem solving or remembering information for short periods. They might find it hard to focus on things which divide attention such as a group conversation, or have problems finding the right word when speaking. These symptoms are known as 'mild cognitive impairment', and at this time, there is no medication offered to help this problem. My search into whether listening to music could affect cognitive ability produced rather mixed results.

Some 25 years ago the media became fascinated with the findings of a study which described how their participants were more successful at cognitive tests set by the researchers after they had listened to Mozart's sonata for two pianos in D major. This became known as the 'Mozart effect' (Rauscher et al 1993). At the time, some parents started playing Mozart to their children in the hope that they would become brighter. Attempts to replicate the study were mixed, though one study by Marzban et al (2011) showed that rats exposed to Mozart had significantly increased brain-derived neurotrophic factor (BDNF) in the hippocampus. BDNF is a protein in the brain which promotes the survival of nerve cells by playing a role in the growth, maturation and maintenance of these cells. In effect, therefore, increasing BDNF encourages a healthy, functioning brain. These rats were young, however, so the Mozart effect might work better on a young brain, but you may wish to listen to the piece and see how it makes you feel. It certainly makes me more alert and I have it playing as I write this! There is other research, too, which suggests that listening to music can help cognition.

A number of studies have shown that listening to music while working can aid episodic memory (Ferreri et al 2013), improve IQ scores (Cockerton et al 1997) verbal and visual processing speed (Angel et al 2010), arithmetic skill (Hallam & Price 1998), reading (Oliver 1997), and learning a second language (Kang & Williamson 2013). The explanation for this improvement is that listening to music affects arousal and mood (Thompson et al 2001) and this in turn affects cognitive ability at that time.

There is research, however, which suggests that background music can *reduce* performance efficiency (Kampfe et al 2010). Not surprisingly, it depends on the type of music, basically whether the tempo is fast or slow, the mode is major or minor, or the music is loud or quiet. A fast tempo in a major key tends to induce a positive/happy mood and higher arousal levels, whereas slow tempo and minor mode music encourages a more negative/sad mood and lower arousal levels (Husain et al 2002). Loud music can interfere with cognitive ability, whereas music played quieter as background can help thinking.

Whether music helps focus also depends on the cognitive demands of the task. For example, background music interfered with surgeons learning a new procedure (Miskovic et al 2008) and people attempting a mathematics task (Bloor 2009). Researchers explain that this is caused by the 'cognitive capacity' theory, which suggests that a limited pool of resources is available for cognitive processing in the brain at any given time and the more complex and demanding the task, the stronger is the detrimental effect of the background music (Furnham & Bradley 1997).

The relationship between music and memory has interested some researchers who have recognised that there is a strong link between emotional music we have heard at specific periods of our lives and our autobiographical memory (Jancke 2008). Researchers have noted that listening to music not only increases blood flow to brain areas involved with emotions (Baumgartner et al 2006), but many other brain areas and the peripheral nervous system (Mizuno & Sugishita 2007). Listening to music activates emotion, memory, attention, imagery etc. in overlapping brain networks. This suggests that the memory-enhancing effect of emotional music might be used to enhance cognitive performance in general. Sarkamo et al (2008) investigated whether listening to music could facilitate the recovery of cognitive functions after a **stroke**. The results showed that verbal memory and focused attention improved significantly in the group of patients who listened to their favourite music daily compared to the patients who listened to audio books or the control group.

There may or may not be a 'Mozart effect' as such but studies have shown that listening to favourite music can have a tremendous influence on our emotional and cognitive system. Furthermore, research into using music as background while you perform another task has shown that the music can have a positive effect on thinking skills and memory if it has a fast enough tempo to lift mood and increase arousal without it being too loud to cause interference and if the task itself isn't too cognitively demanding.

Neurogenesis

Before we leave the subject of the value of listening to music, there is one more potential benefit – neurogenesis, the process by which new neurons are formed in the brain. It used to be thought that the adult brain was fixed and unable to change, but neuroscientists have discovered that neurogenesis occurs not only during embryonic development but can occur in the adult brain too. It has been found to happen in the hippocampi of adult humans and the amygdala (Jhaveri et al 2018).

BDNF has been mentioned earlier in connection with the Mozart effect. BDNF is the main signal that 'turns on' neurogenesis and stimulates neural plasticity (Cortright 2015). One study, which looked at the effect of music compared to noise on the pups of pregnant rats, found that the exposure to music increased neurogenesis in the hippocampus and improved spatial learning ability in the developing rats compared to those which had been exposed to noise (Kim et al 2006). A later study found that exposure to music increased neurogenesis in the motor and somatosensory cortex of the rat pups (Kim et al 2013) If listening to music increases neurogenesis in rats' brains, it seems likely that music could have a similar effect on us.

Chapter summary

- Listening to music can have a strong influence on our mood and our bodies.
- Music can promote 'entrainment', the body's ability to synchronise its rhythms to those of the music being listened to.
- Listening to music produces measurable physiological changes in the body, affecting heart rate, blood pressure, immune system and cortisol levels.
- Slow, relaxing music can help with anxiety, insomnia and pain, while sad music is often preferred by people with depression.
- Listening to music, can reduce the analgesic needed for pain management.
- Music can affect our mood and arousal helping us to focus when doing tasks, if the demands of the task are not too great.

Chapter 3

Moving to music

"Music gives a soul to the universe,
wings to the mind,
flight to the imagination and
life to everything"

PLATO

In the previous chapter we looked at the benefits of simply listening to music. Now, however, it is time to get out of that comfortable chair and to experience the benefits of moving to music. Being able to walk safely and confidently is very important for day to day living and once a person loses this their quality of life diminishes hugely. In this chapter we are going to discover how music can be used to improve gait, its speed and its safety.

Gait problems

Gait problems affect people suffering from various conditions and injuries including multiple sclerosis, cerebral palsy, spinal cord injury and brain injury and we will be looking at the effect of using music to improve walking in these conditions as well as in Parkinson's.

Gait problems are common in Parkinson's, and they interfere with productive movement and safety. As listed in O'Sullivan & Schmitz (2007) the problems can include:

- Flexed or stooped posture when standing and walking
- Decreased range of motion, particularly in hip and knee
- Reduced ankle dorsiflexion
- Decreased trunk and pelvis movement
- Decreased stride length
- Decreased arm swing
- Toe walking with decreased heel strike
- A shuffling gait
- A very slow gait or a fast, festinate gait with increased speed to prevent falling forward
- Difficulty initiating gait
- Freezing
- Difficulty turning or going through doorways
- Poor balance
- Increased cadence (number of steps per minute)
- Decreased velocity (speed)

Many of these problems can lead to an increased susceptibility to falls, which can result in fractures and breakages and even lead to death. Falls are a frequent cause of death in Parkinson's among older patients (Jankovic 2015). Gait problems are generally resistant to medication and are, over time, one of the most incapacitating symptoms for people with Parkinson's (Blin et al 1990). So how can music be used to improve these problems?

Using music as an auditory cue

Very simply, music can provide a cue to stepping. When we dance, we naturally move to the beat and the same can be done in walking. The sound of each musical beat can be a cue to putting the foot to the ground. Using sensory cues to help people with Parkinson's improve their walking was reported as early as 1942 (Von Wilzenben 1942). In the 1960s Trombly noticed that a patient who would freeze severely while walking, did not freeze while dancing to music, and he imagined the possibility of helping a patient function continuously by 'feeding sound into his ears' (Bill 1967).

The first systematic investigations of auditory rhythmic cues in gait training for people with Parkinson's were carried out by Thaut et al (1996) and Miller et al (1996). They found that music, or what they referred to as 'rhythmic auditory stimulation' (RAS) training increased the patient's normal walking speed by as much as 25%, with similar percentage increases in speed of stepping and stride length after only three weeks of training. The authors also found that the patients could walk at their fastest training speed 24 hours after the last training session without a cue, so suggesting the possible effect of a rhythmic entrainment mechanism (entrainment is music's ability to affect the rhythm of the body as seen when we tap our foot to a beat). Most studies into the use of music to benefit gait have measured participants' speed of step, stride length and walking speed at the outset without music, then with music at a comfortable speed. A study the following year by McIntosh et al (1997) suggested that even greater improvements in gait were shown if the rhythmic cues were increased to a speed 10% faster than the participant's baseline speed. These findings are supported in later studies (Howe et al 2003, Arias & Cudeiro 2008).

Suggesting that faster is better has parallels in current research into exercise. The use of exercise to promote the body's own brain repair mechanisms is becoming better understood and recent research has shown that exercise might interfere with multiple mechanisms involved in cell death (Farley et al 2008), stimulate the proliferation of new neurons (Van Pragg 2005), increase blood supply (Kleim et al 2002), and protect against neurodegeneration (Tillerson et al 2002). The exercise, however, needs to be high intensity, involving an 8-out-of-10 self-perceived level of effort (Farley et al 2008). Therefore, walking at a speed 10% faster than comfortable, as well as being a speed which improves gait, also fits the brief for exercise that will benefit the brain.

Baker et al (2008) suggested that because people with Parkinson's have increased gait variability, they will have to pay greater attention during walking than a person without Parkinson's. However, using musical cues reduces gait variability and this suggests that walking to music may reduce the attentional cost of walking. Another study (Hausdorff et al 2007) supports this idea, saying that music enabled more automatic movement with reduced stride-to-stride variability. A study by Willems et al (2007) looked at the ability to turn while walking, something that people with gait problems find challenging, and found that, with music playing, gait-time variability during turning was also reduced.

Many of the researchers tested participants' walking without the musical cue some time after the cued walking test, and they noted a 'carryover' effect. They suggest the possibility of motor plasticity in the parts of the brain controlling rhythmicity. Kadivar et al (2011) found that the carry over benefits of six weeks of walking to music lasted four further weeks.

Participants in another study (De Bruin et al 2010) described the benefits they felt after walking to music.

"I walked with an increased pace, even after turning the music off."

"I stood taller and swung my arms more."

"Exercising was less monotonous."

Freezing, the inability to continue moving forwards, and the fear of freezing have a significant impact on confidence, the desire to go out and quality of life for many with Parkinson's. One study (Arias & Cudeiro 2010) found that patients experienced significantly fewer freezing episodes during the type of walking tasks known to provoke freezing, when they walked to a musical beat that was 10% faster than their baseline walking speed.

Bringing all the study findings together, we note that walking to music increases a Parkinson's patient's step frequency, walking speed and stride length, reduces gait variability, reduces incidents of freezing and falls, makes walking more automatic and improves ability to turn, and these benefits last for some time after the music has stopped. Furthermore, if the beat of the music is 5–10% faster than the baseline walking speed, the improvements in gait are even greater.

Walking to music for other conditions and injuries

Two studies which investigated the effect of music on the walking of **multiple sclerosis** patients (Baram & Millar 2007, Conklyn et al 2010) found significant improvements in step cadence, stride length, step length and walking speed after just one week of walking with music as a cue to stepping.

Several studies (Kwak 2007, Kim et al 2012) have noted how gait performance in **cerebral palsy** can be improved by walking to music. One study (Baram & Lenger 2011) recorded significant improvements in gait parameters in patients with cerebral palsy compared to no change in the gait of the healthy individuals in the control group. This highlights the fact that walking to music does not affect speed *per se*, but rather, for those challenged, it encourages more 'normal' walking.

Patients with **traumatic brain injury** are the focus of a study (Hurt et al 1998) which found that rhythmic auditory stimulation improved their walking speed, step cadence and stride length. And a review of seven studies found walking to music was beneficial for gait improvement in people with **stroke** (Bradt et al 2010).

In the essay, Rhythmic Auditory Stimulation (RAS) Thaut and Rice suggest that **orthopaedic conditions** such as total knee or hip replacement or other joint problems can also benefit from using music to walk to as it will increase weight bearing, range of movement and strength in affected extremities and encourages an even stride between affected and non-affected joints (Thaut & Rice 2014).

What is happening in the brain to cause these improvements in gait?

In previous chapters I have made two important points about the power of music which are relevant here also. Firstly, the body's desire to entrain to music. When we hear music, particularly music with a strong beat, we want to move to it, tap our feet or dance. One researcher explains entrainment:

"The beats found in the music (or auditory stimuli) and the footfalls generated by a gait cycle mark the cycles of the two different oscillatory systems. Through entrainment, the beats and the footfalls get aligned in time" (Moumdjian 2018).

One of the origins of gait impairment in Parkinson's is deficient internal timing (Jones 2008). Another researcher refers to the irregular timing of walking pace as a 'disturbance of coordinated rhythmic locomotion' (Ebersbach et al 1999). An auditory stimulus can provide a regular rhythmic beat to which the body can synchronise.

Studies have tried both visual and tactile cues for walking but auditory is the most successful for two reasons: first, reaction time is 20–50 milliseconds shorter to cues we hear compared to cues we see, and second, the auditory system has a strong bias to detect time-based patterns compared to other sensory systems (Thaut et al 1999).

Music's second important power is its ability to activate many areas of the brain. This means that when the main area controlling movement, the basal ganglia, is compromised, as it is in Parkinson's, another area of the brain, also having the ability to control movement, when activated by the music, can take over. So the intervention of music in Parkinson's alters the activity in the brain's motor and temporal processing networks. According to the authors of a pilot study (Fernández-del-Olmo & Cudeiro 2003), the increased activity they had noted in the cerebellum might mean access to an alternate pathway to compensate for the damaged basal ganglia-SMA-prefrontal cortex path. Other studies support this hypothesis. Debaere et al (2003) notes that externally driven movements in Parkinson's are related to increased activity in the cerebellar-parietal-premotor cortex pathway. And in a report on the neurophysiology of musical cuing using magnetoencephalography, Buard et al (2019) highlights that healthy brains possibly rely on greater frontal mobilisation for auditory entrainment of motor responses, whereas the brains of people with Parkinson's may compensate by using parietal regions.

How to set up a suitable rhythmic auditory cue for walking

Hopefully Parkinson's readers and others with a gait problem will now be keen to see if walking to music benefits them. However, please only try walking to music if you are safe to do so or if you have the assistance of a therapist, carer or friend who will keep you safe.

First, it is very important that you choose music at a suitable speed for you. Two studies by Brown et al (Brown et al 2009, 2010) researched the effect on gait of people with Parkinson's who listened to music while they walked but did not choose music with either a strong beat or at an appropriate tempo. In both studies, gait and obstacle crossing were adversely affected because, rather than synchronising with the movement, the music was providing an added cognitive challenge.

Before downloading music to walk to, you will first need to determine the speed which corresponds with your step cadence (the number of steps you walk per minute). To do this you will initially need a portable metronome. If you have a smartphone you could download a metronome app. Alternatively a digital metronome is relatively inexpensive to purchase and light enough to be carried. A metronome is used in music to set the speed for a piece and marks the number of beats per minute. I suggest you calculate your preferred walking speed by the trial and error method.

Initially, set the metronome at a speed somewhere from 80–110 beats per minute (bpm), 80 bpm if you are a slow walker, 110 bpm if you are fit. Listen to the beat for a minute or two and then start walking on a flat path, making sure you step in time to the metronome ticks. Walk about 20–30 yards to decide whether the speed is too fast or too slow for you. Adjust up or down by increments of 5 bpm until you find your most comfortable speed.

The next task is to choose suitable music for your walking playlist. Some suggestions are included in the appendices at the back of the book at various walking speeds. The music must have a STRONG low disco style beat, i.e. 'foot tapping' music. Classical music or easy-listening style recordings do not work for this. However, your children and grandchildren will be very impressed at your song choice! Although I would never actually sit and listen to my walking playlist, as it is not my preferred style of music to listen to, it is perfect for walking. The music also needs to be played loud enough so that you feel part of the music, without damaging your hearing. Lastly you will need lightweight or earbud headphones to provide music loud enough without disturbing fellow walkers.

Once you have chosen your music (you can download it from a music-streaming service, like Spotify, Tidal, Apple Music, Qobuz, Primephone, Amazon Music Limited, Deezer or YouTube Music, or buy it from iTunes etc.), make a playlist on your smart phone or iPod so that your music is portable, and plug in your headphones.

You are now ready to head off, along your selected path, stepping in time to the beat of the music, while making sure the heel of your foot touches the path with each beat. How far you walk will depend on your fitness. If you are not a frequent walker, begin with a ten-minute walk and gradually increase the distance as you are able. I like to walk for 45 minutes now, though I began at ten minutes when I started using walking as an exercise five years ago.

The research reports that stride and speed of walking increased in the studies using this method, so it is possible that your preferred walking speed may change over time. Many of the studies increased the speed their participants walked after a set period and found that asking people to walk with cues that were 5–10% faster in tempo than their baseline cadence produced even greater improvements on gait deficits. As mentioned earlier, the exercise needs to be 'effortful'.

Instead of music, some studies have used a single sound, like a regular tick or click, or a metronome to define the beat. Although these studies have seen improvements to gait by this method of auditory stimulus, burying the beat within music is better. The components of music, the pitch and rhythm combining to produce melody, help us to anticipate when the next beat is coming and of course, music is more enjoyable to listen to than a tick!

Some researchers considered whether people with Parkinson's, rather than *listening* to music, could sing mentally while walking to improve their gait (Satoh & Kuzuhara 2008). The participants were trained over seven progressive tasks towards being able to walk while mentally singing. After just a single session of training, the participants' speed and stride length improved significantly and participants reported that they had successfully used mental singing in their daily lives.

I accept that singing mentally is more convenient than going to the trouble of recording a playlist. However, I feel that mental singing is not a substitute for walking to a recording of music. The beat of recorded music drives you on providing entrainment, whereas when mentally singing, without an outside beat, you are more likely to adapt your singing to suit your walking, rather than adapting the walking to keep with a regular beat. You are also unlikely to increase the speed, as was recommended earlier. However, if the tools of recorded music are unavailable, or you are walking short distances, around the house for example, then singing mentally does offer an alternative. If you try this, pick a song which you can mentally sing at the same speed as your preferred walking speed. Soldiers often sing as they march, and a marching song would be a reasonable choice. It is also worth trying mental singing in an emergency, if you find yourself freezing for example.

Dance

A chapter on moving to music would not be complete without talking about dance. Of course, the special influences that music has, which make walking easier for a person with Parkinson's, will also make dance moves easier. However, whereas studies on cued walking have measured the particular effect of the music on the activity, no study has compared dancing with music to dancing without. Studies have been more interested in the effect of the particular physical movement and style of dance.

Studies into dance-based rehabilitation in Parkinson's disease have noted muscle-coordination improvements (Allen et al 2017) and increases in comfortable and fast-as-possible walking speed, step speed and balance (Hackney & Earhart 2009). One case study (Hackney & Earhart 2010) followed an individual with severe Parkinson's who used a wheelchair and found that after twenty partnered tango lessons, his balance, endurance, confidence and quality of life had improved. Dance requires a dynamic pattern of stops, starts, turns, side-steps and backward walking depending on the particular dance style and this may explain why balance improvements are noted in the majority of dance studies on Parkinson's patients.

Joining a dance group is beneficial for anyone and particularly worth considering for someone with Parkinson's. As well as the physical exercise, it provides an opportunity for socialising and can lift mood. However, while you are doing your Irish fling or your tango, spare a thought for the power of music. The physical exertion and body movements are very beneficial to brain and body but remember that music is really the unsung hero. It is music that is making the control of your movements easier.

Motivation and fatigue

Before we leave the subject of this chapter – moving to an auditory stimulus – I want to highlight two further gifts which scientists have found music gives us: motivation to exercise and reduced feelings of fatigue during exercise.

As mentioned earlier, several studies point to exercise having a neuroprotective effect on the brain (Bayod et al 2011, Tajiri et al 2009) through encouraging an increase of BDNF (Ahlskog 2011) and producing improvement in deteriorated motor function. Anything which encourages exercise, therefore, is worth considering. One recent study found that using music to exercise to increased arousal and perceived enjoyment to a greater degree than listening to a podcast or listening to nothing (Costas et al 2019). Studies have also suggested that music can distract the listener who is exercising from feelings of fatigue (Lim et al 2011).

Having the ability and the confidence to walk is fundamental to basic functioning and quality of life. Music can improve all gait parameters, making walking easier, safer and more enjoyable. Furthermore, movement and exercise are very important in Parkinson's for the benefits it provides body and brain, and music can motivate involvement in this exercise.

Chapter summary

- This chapter has pointed to many ways in which music can help movement.
- It can stimulate alternative neural motor pathways in the brains of people with Parkinson's whose normal motor function is restricted.
- It provides entrainment, giving the body a rhythm with which to synchronise movement.
- Walking to music at 5–10% more than a comfortable walking speed improves gait: encouraging less gait variability, increasing walking speed, step stride, arm swing, improving turning, reducing falls and freezing. These improvements will continue when walking without music.
- Using music to walk to has also been shown to improve gait in other conditions including multiple sclerosis, cerebral palsy, traumatic brain injury, stroke and orthopaedic conditions.
- Music can motivate people to exercise and distract them from feelings of fatigue.

Chapter 4

Making music

"Music... will help dissolve your perplexities and
purify your character and sensibilities,
and in time of care and sorrow,
will keep a fountain of joy alive in you."

DIETRICH BONHOEFFER

Eating lunch with my brother recently, he told me what he did to stay healthy and said "What more can I do?" Slightly tongue in cheek I told him to hum and sing, for humming and singing have many benefits for everyone.

In earlier chapters we have considered listening to and moving to music. It is now time to make some music ourselves. This chapter will explore how singing, humming and playing a musical instrument can have tremendous benefits for brain, body and mood, as well as improving symptoms affecting people with Parkinson's and other conditions.

Before we explore the benefits of singing identified by published research, I would like first to consider breathing. After all, we need to breathe before we can sing or speak, and various studies have pointed to the significant benefits of deep breathing.

Intentional breathing

Apparently we usually breathe between 10–20 times per minute (Russo et al 2017) which adds up to 15–30,000 or more breaths per day. It is fortunate that we do not have to remember to breathe to keep ourselves alive as I am not sure how successful we would be. However, the act of controlling breathing in a particular way to enhance health has been practised for thousands of years, particularly among Eastern cultures (Russo et al 2017). Yoga has several different breathing practices called 'pranayama'. But what actually happens when we breathe?

Breathing has two phases, inspiration and expiration. During inspiration the diaphragm and the external intercostal muscles (the muscles that run between our ribs) contract. The diaphragm moves downward which increases the volume of the chest cavity, and the external intercostal muscles pull the ribs up and outward, which causes the rib-cage to expand and the chest volume to increase further. This increase in volume lowers the air pressure in the lungs compared to atmospheric air, and because air always flows from an area of high pressure to one of low pressure, air comes in through the mouth or nose, then moves through the throat, larynx and trachea into the lungs. During the expiration phase, the diaphragm and external intercostal muscles relax, returning the chest cavity to its smaller volume and forcing the air out of the lungs.

There are many benefits of slow deep breathing, one of which, **reducing stress,** is often studied. One study, published in the *International Journal of Yoga* (Naik et al 2018) found that after 12 weeks of slow breathing exercise training, the study participants' heart rate, blood pressure, and perceived stress had decreased significantly. A study of nursing students by Consolo et al (2008) used diaphragmatic breathing to reduce their anxiety prior to examinations. The breathing exercises successfully reduced heart rates and improved exam performance. Tomokolnoue (2012) found that deep breathing intervention was likely to reduce the tension, anxiety and fatigue in patients undergoing chemotherapy, and Perciavalle et al (2016), using mood and stress evaluation charts as well as measuring heart rate and salivary cortisol, found that using a deep breathing technique was effective in improving mood and stress.

One study (Martarelli et al 2011) monitored sixteen athletes during an exhaustive training session for the effects of diaphragmatic breathing on exercise-induced oxidative stress and the roles of **cortisol** and **melatonin** hormones on this stress pathway. Results showed that deep breathing increased the antioxidant defence status in athletes after exhaustive exercise by decreasing cortisol and increasing melatonin.

Zaccaro et al (2018) studied the physiological effects of deep breathing. They found that slow breathing promotes autonomic changes, increasing **heart rate variability** (the variation in time between heart beats, with a higher HRV indicating better health) and **respiratory sinus arrhythmia** (HRV in synchrony with respiration) and alpha (the resting state for the brain) and decreasing theta power. They identified that this led to increased comfort, relaxation, vigour and alertness with reduced arousal, anxiety, depression, anger and confusion.

Pain processing has also been found to be affected by deep breathing. Busch et al's (2012) results suggested that deep, slow breathing reduced sympathetic nervous system arousal and pain perception. Deep breathing has also been found effective for reducing **depression** (Chung 2010).

People with **Chronic Obstructive Pulmonary Disease** (COPD) can benefit from deep breathing exercises. Fernandes et al (2011) found that it can improve the breathing pattern and ventilatory efficiency without causing dyspnea (shortness of breath) in patients whose respiratory muscular system is preserved. Cooper et al (2003) suggests deep breathing is also good for other pulmonary diseases such as asthma.

Further studies have identified deep breathing as benefitting **hypertension** (Chodzinski 2000), **post-traumatic stress disorder** (PTSD) (Kim et al 2013), **irritable bowel syndrome** (IBS) (Lakhan & Schofield 2013) and **insomnia** (Ong et al 2014).

Respiration problems in Parkinson's

Many of the health issues listed above, such as anxiety depression, insomnia and fatigue, are experienced by Parkinson's patients. However, many Parkinson's patients also mention other breathing challenges. One study (Lee et al 2007), measuring the symptom load in Parkinson's, found that 35.8% reported shortness of breath on exertion (dyspnea), 17.9% reported a cough and 13% reported phlegm production. Pennington et al (2010) reported that a higher proportion of Parkinson's patients die of pneumonia than in the general population. Hypoxia, when the body has insufficient oxygen and hypercapnia, a build-up of carbon dioxide in the bloodstream, can happen when breathing is not adequate. There is also a chance of increased respiratory infections. Upper airway obstruction has been reported in a third of people with Parkinson's, the most common manifestation of which is soft speech which affects as many as 70% of people with the disease (Torsney & Forsyth 2017). Many people with Parkinson's produce more variable and less efficient movements of the chest wall when preparing to speak, taking in less breath before speaking and continuing to speak when breath reserves were finished (Bunton 2005).

Patients themselves are frequently unaware that their speech is accelerating or slurred or unclear, and frequently complain that it is their partner who is becoming deaf. This denial is referred to as 'anosognosia' (Prigatano et al 2010).

Researchers have suggested various causes for breathing problems in Parkinson's. Baille et al (2018) identified inspiratory muscle weakness, even in early-stage patients. Rigidity, a common symptom of Parkinson's, can affect the muscles of the chest wall and the diaphragm, which will restrict the movement needed to breathe fully. Furthermore, a stooped posture, affecting many, can reduce lung volume. Torsney & Forsyth (2017) further suggest that the reduction in dopamine of the condition itself may cause shortness of breath or the perception of shortness of breath. Breathing is driven by high carbon dioxide and low oxygen levels in the blood, which is regulated by the brainstem and carotid bodies respectively. The loss of dopaminergic input to the brainstem and carotid bodies can cause altered regulation of the carbon dioxide and oxygen and consequently an altered perception of breathing.

Suggested breathing practices

Breathing exercises will help to improve all conditions mentioned. There are many different breathing practices, some designed to waken while others aim to relax. Two of the simpler ones will be described here. Both are relaxing and quite adequate for achieving all the benefits previously discussed. YouTube has many other breathing practices.

These exercises can be practised lying down or sitting upright but don't try them straight after a meal! It is important to be relaxed and be able to fully expand both ribcage and abdomen. Tight clothes may need to be loosened. One hand should be placed on the abdomen and the other on the upper chest. This will provide a way of checking whether breathing is deep enough. On taking in a deep breath, the hand on the abdomen should rise (if lying down), while the hand on the upper chest should not move. To check whether the ribcage is expanding, the hand on the upper chest can be moved to the side. Then as the breathing exercise is practiced both the hand on the abdomen and the hand on the side of the ribcage should show movement.

Breathing exercise 1:
Breathe in deeply through the nose, expanding abdomen and ribcage to a slow count of 5, and out for a slow count of 5. Repeat for 7–10 minutes.

Or

Breathing exercise 2:
Breathe in deeply through the nose, expanding abdomen and ribcage to a count of 4, hold for a count of 4 and exhale for a slow count of 6–8. Repeat for 7–10 minutes.

It is important in both these exercises that you stay relaxed. If you start to tense, it may be because you are counting slower than you can currently manage.

Singing

Having learnt how to take a deep breath, we are now ready to sing. Singing is a valuable therapeutic tool because it is a universal form of musical expression that is as natural as speaking. It is found in every culture and age. Even babies produce vocalisations which are precursors for music and singing.

There was a time when, if we wanted to hear music, we made it ourselves, be it at school, in church, alone or together. However, in our modern world it is as though we have been silenced, unprepared to sing in public for fear of being judged. Many of us have been told we cannot sing. What is more, we compare ourselves to the carefully produced recordings of our idols and our lack of confidence plummets further. Yet singing provides many health benefits for all of us. We need to sing for the good of our brain, our body and our mood and the good news is that you do not have to have a good voice to reap the benefits.

How do our brains and bodies produce sound? In both singing and speaking, during an out breath, the air goes through the larynx and causes the vocal folds in the larynx to vibrate. These vibrations make the sound, with the shape of a person's nose, mouth and throat giving each voice its individuality. The muscles in the larynx contract to change the pitch of the voice.

There are several small differences between the mechanics of speech and singing. With singing there is a larger tidal volume of air used. Speaking generally uses lower frequency levels (pitch) and a narrower range of frequencies. Also, the vowel to consonant duration rate is less in speaking, roughly 5:1 and greater in singing, ranging up to 200:1. The brain's involvement differs too. When we speak, the left hemisphere, which controls word formation and sentence structure, is involved. But when we sing, the right hemisphere, where rhythm and melody is produced, takes over, which explains why speech impediments like stuttering largely disappear when the person sings.

General health benefits of singing

Many of the benefits of singing come from the slower than normal respiration required, and the health benefits already mentioned for breathing apply also, therefore, to singing. Various studies, though, have suggested further benefits.

Several studies have considered the self-reported benefits of singing in a choir (Moss et al 2017, Daykin et al 2017, Judd & Pooley 2013). Clift and Hancox (2001) surveyed members of a university college choral society and found that 87% said they benefitted socially, 75% emotionally and 58% physically. The health benefits which the participants highlighted were improved lung function and breathing, improved mood and stress reduction and benefits for heart and immune system. Clift (2010) headed a team of researchers who looked at the psychological wellbeing of choral singers, sending questionnaires to over 600 members of choirs in England. They found that most singers found the effects of singing positive in terms of perceived enhancement of well-being. The questionnaires invited the participants to write comments and many said that choral singing engendered happiness and raised spirits which counteracted feelings of sadness and depression, and that the deep controlled breathing for singing counteracted anxiety. They also suggested that choral singing offered social support and friendship, reducing any feelings of isolation and loneliness. The average age of the singers questioned was 61 and it was not surprising that they also identified that learning songs kept their minds active and counteracted any decline of cognitive function.

Two other studies have also researched singing for older people. Houston et al (1998) reported significant reductions in levels of anxiety and depression in nursing home residents following a four-week programme of singing. Cohen et al (2006) found significant improvements in both the mental and physical health of a group of elderly people after a year attending a community choir.

'Singing your heart out could make you happier', is the title of a 2017 study (Shakespeare & Whieldon 2017) which found that people who took part in a community singing group maintained or improved their mental health. The combination of singing and socialising was an essential part of recovery from mental problems because it promoted an ongoing feeling of belonging and wellbeing.

Some studies have looked for quantitative, physiological evidence of the effect of singing on the body. A study by Fancourt et al (2016) found that just one hour singing in a choir, boosted **levels of immune proteins** in people affected by cancer, **stress** was reduced and mood improved, which in turn could have a positive impact on overall health. The study tested 193 choir members of different choirs and found that an hour's singing significantly reduced stress hormones, such as cortisol, and increased quantities of cytokines, proteins of the immune system, which can boost the body's ability to fight serious illness. The findings supported an earlier study by Kreutz et al (2004) which found that singing in a choir boosted the immune system and decreased cortisol to a greater extent than when merely listening to music.

A study (Keeler et al 2015) into the neurochemistry of singing found that group singing reduced stress and arousal, and increased oxytocin, a hormone which is sometimes known as the 'love hormone' because it is released when people cuddle or when they bond socially. Oxytocin has been found to alleviate anxiety and stress. A more recent study (Schladt et al 2017) compared the effect of 20 minutes solo singing compared to 20 minutes choral singing on oxytocin and cortisol levels. The results showed that both situations increased happiness and decreased sadness and worry as measured by oxytocin and cortisol levels, but found that the positive effects were more pronounced after choir singing compared to solo singing. Lastly, a study by Pearce et al (2015) compared the bonding experience of three new groups, singing, craft and creative writing, and found that although all groups felt equally connected at the end of seven months, the singers had bonded the quickest.

Singing can help **pain**. Dunbar et al (2012) measured endorphin release using pain threshold as a test. Endorphins are neurotransmitters which transmit electrical signals within the central nervous system. Endorphins interact with the opiate receptors in the brain to reduce our perception of pain and act in a similar way to drugs such as morphine and codeine. They also help to promote positive feelings. The study found that singing, dancing and drumming all triggered endorphin release more efficiently than simply listening to music.

Singing also improves depression. Many women suffer from **postnatal depression** in the first 40 weeks post-birth. A study by Fancourt and Perkins (2018), divided 134 mothers into a singing group, a mothers and babies play group and a control group. After ten weeks, the mothers in the singing group showed the fastest improvement from postnatal depression.

Singing also works as an exercise to strengthen the throat and palate muscles. This can have huge benefits for people with snoring and sleep apnea problems, as well as dysarthria and dysphagia, common symptoms in Parkinson's.

Snoring is caused by pharyngeal narrowing or collapse, which leads to a reduction in or stopping of airflow during sleep which causes the loud breathing noise. Sedatives, prescription sleeping tablets and alcohol can all cause this because they reduce muscle tone in the upper airways and pharynx, which leads to the airways narrowing. If snoring deteriorates it can lead to the more serious condition of **sleep apnea**.

Hilton et al (2013) conducted a study which recruited 93 people with a history of snoring and sleep apnea dividing them between a study group and control group. The study group were given recordings of singing exercises and asked to perform them for 20 minutes daily. The researchers found that daily singing for 20 minutes over a three month period improved the tone and strength of pharyngeal muscles and this in turn reduced the severity, frequency and loudness of snoring and improved the symptoms of mild to moderate sleep apnea.

Singing has been found to reduce **stuttering**. Healey et al (1976) asked participants to read and to sing the lyrics of well-known songs. The reduction in stuttering was greater in the singing than the reading condition. Andrews et al (1982) found that singing reduced the frequency of stuttering by over 90%, which they thought was caused by the longer syllables in singing. Glover et al (1996) compared singing and reading at slow and fast rate and found no difference in stuttering frequency between the two different 'speed' conditions but noted a 75% reduction in stuttering when the participants were instructed to sing. The authors point out that there was no claim that the participants were all actually singing, as capabilities varied greatly, but they found that just the instruction to sing led to the huge improvements.

Precisely why singing is a good therapeutic tool for stuttering has been largely unexplored, though various hypotheses have been suggested. One is that continuous voicing helps to increase the connectedness between syllables and words (Andrews et al 1982). While Ozdemir et al (2006) found that although both hemispheres of the brain are involved in speaking and singing, stuttering is more connected to the left hemisphere which is more involved with speech, while singing shows more activation of the right hemisphere.

Benefits of singing for Parkinson's

Speech problems in Parkinson's have been mentioned previously in connection with inadequate breathing, and this is certainly one origin, but speech problems are also caused by lack of muscle tone in the throat and palate. **Dysarthria** is the term used for difficult or unclear articulation of speech which is otherwise linguistically normal. It is a neurological motor speech impairment characterised by

- a softer, breathy, or hoarse voice known as hypophonia,
- slurred speech,
- a voice that is monotonal in pitch, lacking the normal ups and downs, with the upper part of the frequency range lost (Viallet et al 2000)
- lacking prosody: intonation, tone, stress and rhythm and having inappropriate pauses
- short rushes of speech and a variable rate (Darley et al 1969)

There are many causes for the speech challenges in Parkinson's including neural pathway problems which affect motor control, muscle atrophy, particularly in the larynx, muscle rigidity in all components used in speech including the mask-like face and rigidity of mouth, tongue and jaw, and lastly insufficient intake of breath and breath control.

During the progression of Parkinson's disease, over 70% of people mention that their speech is impaired (Miller et al 2006), which can lead to social isolation (Karlsen et al 2000). In a survey of 460 Parkinson's and multiple sclerosis patients, 44% of the multiple sclerosis patients had also experienced speech impairment (Hartelius & Svensson 1994). Twenty-nine percent of Parkinson's patients and 16% of multiple sclerosis patients regarded the speech disorder as one of their greatest problems and yet only 3% of Parkinson's and 2% of the multiple sclerosis patients had received speech therapy. Dysarthria is also a frequent problem for people with brain tumours and for the elderly, especially those who live alone and who use their voice infrequently during the day.

Often people with dysarthria may also have **dysphagia**, which is the inefficient or unsafe transfer of food, liquid or saliva from mouth to stomach. One dysphagia problem is a delay in triggering the swallow action (Yorkston et al 2004). Serious complications of dysphagia can include aspiration pneumonia, malnutrition and dehydration. In the survey of 460 patients, 41% of Parkinson's patients and 33% of multiple sclerosis patients indicated that they had problems chewing or swallowing (Hartelius & Svensson 1994).

Both singing and swallowing affect similar muscles and several studies have considered the feasibility of singing in a choir as a therapy for speech and swallowing problems. Improvements noted in these studies include significant changes in singing quality and voice range with no decline in speaking quality over time (Elefant et al 2012), increases in intensity, range and pitch (Tanner 2016), improved respiratory pressure (Stegemoller et al 2017), greater tongue excursion during vowel articulation with increased speech intelligibility (Higgins et al 2019), and improvements in vocal intensity and maximum expiratory pressure (Tamplin et al 2019). Haneishi (2001) used a music-based voice programme which consisted of voice warm-ups and singing exercises, emphasising articulation and breathing and participants showed significant increases in clarity and volume of speech after 12–14 sessions.

Few studies have looked into any specific exercises for swallowing problems though there are several in use with some wonderful names including 'the effortful swallow', 'Mendelsohn', 'super-supraglottic', 'Masako' and the 'McNeill dysphagia treatment protocol'. There are also some exercises which do not specifically concentrate on swallowing in the exercise like Shaker head lift, tongue strengthening, and the Lee Silverman voice treatment and expiratory muscle strength training, which concentrates on strengthening the force of the out breath by using a device you blow into (Langmore & Pisegna 2015). The aims of each technique focus on different components of the swallow action. The little research there is into any of these exercises, however, tends to be small scale and often uses healthy participants.

Singing and swallowing both use the laryngeal muscles. Different vocal fold movements are required for various laryngeal functions (Ludlow 2005). The vocal folds are open the most during a sniff, open during inhalation, less open during exhalation, closed in the midline during voice production, elongated for high-pitched singing, tightly closed for a cough, and there is sphincteric closure of both the vocal and ventricular folds during swallowing. Because singing and swallowing both use the laryngeal muscles, singing has been found to improve swallowing. Stegemoller et al (2017) gave 24 Parkinson's patients eight weeks of group singing. Electromyography (EMG) was used to measure the muscle activity associated with swallow before and after the singing intervention. Results showed a significant increase in EMG outcome measures. The researchers suggested that singing prolonged the time the larynx was elevated, a movement which strengthened the muscles used to protect the airway from foreign material during the swallow. In various studies, Parkinson's and stroke participants also reported quality of life improvements; improvement in mood (Fogg-Rogers et al 2014), and social support and emotional well-being (Irons et al 2018).

A non-music-based intensive voice programme, known as the Lee Silverman voice treatment (LSVT), named after the first person treated and based on loud phonation and high intensity vocal exercises while emphasising breathing, has been seen to be effective in reducing some of the speech abnormalities experienced by patients with Parkinson's. However, the programme has limitations in its availability, its high cost related to the intensity of required client contact time and the significant numbers who drop out for one reason or another (Matthews et al 2018). Group singing as a comparison therapy, is inexpensive, has high availability and participation uptake, low drop-out and provides social support for its participants.

How to improve speech and swallow problems

Before you embark on a programme of therapeutic singing it might be a good idea to make an audio or video recording of how your speaking voice currently sounds. You may be surprised at how quiet you sound, how limited your pitch range is or how little you move your mouth. Don't be too disappointed, as including singing in your daily schedule will soon produce improvements and another recording in a few months should show this.

There are several ways in which singing can be incorporated into your life. You can join a choir. Community choirs which welcome all comers without auditions are becoming very popular. You will benefit more quickly if you also sing several times at home between choir sessions. To do this you could sing along to one of the many vocal warm-up videos on YouTube, or you could make a playlist of your favourite songs and sing along with them. I like to sing with Barbra Streisand. Keeping the volume of Barbra up gives me the confidence to sing out! You could also sing along with the radio. Remember, it does not matter what you sound like. You are not doing this to become a pop star or sing at La Scala Milan. You are doing it to speak more confidently and to swallow more safely.

Humming

Before we leave the subject of voiced music making, we will have a quick look at the benefits of humming, making a noise while keeping the lips closed. If you are doing it correctly, the 'hum' will stop if you pinch your nose closed.

When we hum we slow our breathing down, as we do when singing. The 12–20 breaths per minute we take normally can reduce to 4–6 breaths per minute when we hum, and the benefits noted for deep breathing, i.e. reduced blood pressure, heart rate, anxiety, depression, insomnia, fatigue and pain, are also encouraged by humming. Some forms of meditation incorporate humming in the form of 'OM' to help calm the mind and the body. In a brain imaging study (Kalyani et al 2011), the meditation chant 'OM', where the Mmmmm part of 'om' is continued, reduced activity in areas of the brain associated with **depression**. The researchers speculated that vibrations from the OM chanting may have stimulated the vagus nerve, which then sent out electrical signals that deactivated key areas of the brain connected with depression.

Humming benefits the **sinuses** because it increases nasal nitric oxide. A study by Weltzberg et al (2002) found that nitric oxide in the nose increased 15-fold during humming compared to quiet breath exhalations. Nitric oxide is known to be broadly antifungal, antiviral and antibacterial. One case report (Eby 2006) monitored a subject with chronic rhinosinusitis who hummed strongly at a low pitch for one hour daily. After four days the symptoms had largely been eliminated. Coincidentally, his cardiac arrhythmias were also greatly lessened.

Although humming for an hour at a time is quite excessive, five or ten minutes is manageable and should be productive. After a deep breath, hum on a single note/pitch for a count of eight or ten. You will probably feel pleasant vibrations in your face and head. Experiment with long notes on different pitches. Alternatively you may like to hum a favourite tune.

Rhythmic cueing for speech

A further way in which music can be used as a therapeutic tool for speech is by using the tick of a metronome as a rhythmic cue. Where the speech problem is slurred or unclear articulation, this can slow the rate of speech down, giving time to coordinate articulatory muscles, while providing a stable time anchor to which the patient can adjust. Mainka and Mallien discuss the use of rhythmic speech cueing (RSC) in music therapy in the *Handbook of Neurologic Music Therapy*, (Mainka & Mallien 2014), noting that it is effective for dysarthria in patients with Parkinson's disease. Furthermore, Parkinson's patients have a tendency to speed up (known as 'festination') when performing repetitive movements. This festination has been discussed in the previous chapter in connection with gait but it can also disturb handwriting and speech. Interestingly, in Parkinson's patients it is mainly seen in those with left-sided symptom dominance (Flasskamp et al 2012). Tripoliti et al (2011) suggest that deep brain stimulation can make oral festination worse. Speaking to a rhythmic cue seems to help regulate the speaking pace in Parkinson's. It offers rhythmic entrainment, which facilitates a better motor programming for the process of speaking, similar to the way in which a musical beat helps the gross motor functions of walking discussed in Chapter 3.

Rhythmic cueing can also offer a treatment for **stuttering** (Ingham et al 2009) and helps speech in **post-stroke patients** (Brendel & Ziegler 2008).

How to use rhythmic cueing

To try rhythmic cueing, you will need a means of recording, a metronome and something to read. Firstly, record your voice as you read a paragraph at your normal speed. Secondly, set your metronome to a slow speed. I suggest about 150 bpm to begin with. Normal speech rates in reading range between 200–360 syllables per minute and rhythmic cueing was found to be most effective at 60% of this speed (Thaut et al 2001). Thirdly, read one syllable to each metronome tick while consciously exaggerating your mouth and tongue movements as you read to encourage new habits of clearer enunciation and speaking loudly. I suggest practising for 5–10 minutes each day for a week and then re-recording yourself speaking or reading normally without the cue. Note any improvements, however small and continue practising daily and recording weekly.

Playing an instrument

The easy availability of recorded music has not lessened the demand for instrumental lessons among adults, even if schools are reducing their emphasis on class music and the availability of peripatetic instrument tuition. The satisfaction of producing ordered sounds, recognisable as a known tune, is still hugely rewarding for many.

Playing a musical instrument is an excellent rehabilitative tool too, offering opportunities to benefit body, brain and mood. For the body, playing any instrument works the arms, hands and fingers of the upper body requiring both gross and fine motor movements. For the brain, playing any instrument employs multiple components of the central and peripheral nervous system. The player uses motor systems in the brain to control the gross and fine movements needed to make the sound. The sound is processed by the auditory circuit, while sensory information from fingers, hands and arms is sent to the brain for processing. If the player is using music, then visual information is also sent to the brain for interpreting before commands are sent to the motor centres. The player also emotionally interprets the sounds and, at times, coordinates with other instrumentalists (Zatorre et al 2007).

Motor function has been shown to benefit from various different therapeutic strategies (Quinn et al 2013, Mateos-Toset et al 2015). However, I would like to suggest five reasons why playing a musical instrument offers the best method for strengthening upper extremities and improving independence of arms, hands and fingers, with many advantages over other forms of upper body exercise.

Firstly, the five core principles of motor learning are met when playing an instrument. Repetition is employed when a piece is practised and the music provides a satisfactory purpose to the task. The activity provides feedback. It is possible to graduate the complexity of the activity and the music produced supplies motivation for the exercise.

Secondly, playing an instrument is one of the few exercises that provides auditory as well as kinaesthetic feedback. The auditory feedback from the instrument together with the entrainment caused by the rhythmic cues create a feedback loop. The performer knows what sound s/he should be producing, and this enables the player to plan, anticipate and execute his/her movements in a more efficient way.

Thirdly, playing an instrument can have a positive effect on mood. The music produced can calm, lift spirits and ease depression. It can provide an opportunity for creativity and self-expression and can provide motivation to keep going (Pacchetti et al 2000). I asked my piano pupils what they got out of learning and practising the piano. They told me it made them happy and took them away from everyday problems. One said, "*The satisfaction and sense of accomplishment I experience when I manage to recreate, even partially, a piece of music that I like, is immense.*"

Fourthly, long-term music making, either practising an instrument or singing, can bring about plastic changes in the brain (Gaser & Schlaug 2003). Salimpoor et al (2013) gives support to the idea that musical practice may be the perfect tool for neuro-education and rehabilitation because it encourages plastic changes both in the healthy and the damaged brain. It is certainly a full body workout for the brain, involving multiple areas simultaneously, integrating information from the senses of vision, hearing and touch.

Musicians have served as a unique model for studying plastic changes in the human brain because of the complexity of this single stimulus. Studies with musicians who have practiced more than 10,000 hours (Krampe & Ericsson 1996) before they became professional have shown the resulting neuroplastic changes (Kolbe & Mohammod 2014). One area which shows change is the hippocampus, which is involved in learning and memory. Neurogenesis, the formation of new neurons, is a critical process for learning and memory in the hippocampus, and Hyde et al (2009) suggest that musical practice may therefore enhance neurogenesis, thereby leading to improved learning and memory activity. Bengtsson et al (2005) investigated the brain's white matter which is made mostly of myelin and surrounds the axons of neurons and increases the speed of nerve impulses. They found that white matter was enhanced by practising the piano, particularly in the corpus callosum, the white matter that connects the two hemispheres of the brain. Francois et al (2015) and Rodrigues et al (2010) provide reviews of many more studies identifying the neuroplastic effect of musical training on the brain.

Fifthly, music-making activities can also bring about the establishment of alternative neural pathways in the brain, which can circumvent dysfunctional brain regions in neurogenerative disorders (Wan et al 2010). Thaut's work has been discussed in chapter three; his concept of 'entrainment', the idea that stimulating the portion of the brain that perceives sound and rhythm, can also synchronise other areas of the brain, including the region responsible for movement.

People with Parkinson's frequently experience diminishing manual dexterity (Proud & Morris 2010) and muscle weakness (Allen et al 2009), caused through bradykinesia (slowness of movement), rigidity and tremor. This affects the ability to carry out everyday activities such as handwriting, buttoning and tying shoelaces, which impacts on quality of life. Some studies have reported upper limb problems predominantly affecting one side or the other, including delayed onset in opening the hand, delayed initiation of the forearm movement, lack of coordination, loss of muscle control and difficulties in the independence between left and right arm (Tuelings et al 1997). Decreased physical activity, however, is not only a *symptom* of Parkinson's but may also increase the underlying degeneration (Tillerson et al 2002). Understandably it is easier to use a strong limb to carry out a task, but this learnt non-use can exacerbate the problem, while forced use and continuous practice with the weaker limb can preserve existing abilities, retard progression of symptoms and possibly reverse motor impairments (Fisher et al 2004). I came across a saxophone player who changed to playing a trombone because his fingers were weakened through Parkinson's and fingers are not used individually when playing a trombone. Although this might have been more satisfying musically, it was less useful therapeutically.

If playing an instrument is to be a therapeutic activity, then consideration needs to be given to the physical requirements needed to produce a sound, as each instrument varies. Brass and woodwind instruments use breath to make a sound, so slow, deep breathing, with all the benefits already mentioned, is needed. Although woodwind instruments, like flute, clarinet and saxophone use the fingers of both hands, brass instruments, such as trumpet, trombone and tuba, with only three or four valves to depress, tend to exercise only the fingers of one hand. A stringed instrument, such as violin, cello or double bass, while employing the fingers of the left hand to stop the strings to produce the correct note, requires little individual right hand finger work apart from balancing and guiding the bow. So if you are hoping to exercise the fingers of both hands because of current limitations due to a neurodegenerative disorder or the stiffness and swelling of arthritis, for example, woodwind instruments, the harp, the guitar and keyboard instruments would be the most suitable.

Playing a musical instrument can help cognitive as well as motor problems. A study by Vik et al (2018) explored the effects of playing the piano on patients with cognitive impairment after **mild traumatic brain injury** (mTBI), investigating whether this approach would stimulate neural networks to rerouting neural connections and linking up cortical circuits that had been disrupted. After just eight weeks playing piano, the patients with mTBI, who had had attention, memory and social interaction problems, showed improved cognitive performance.

Choosing an instrument

It would be difficult to make suggestions as to which instrument should be played when readers could include everyone from the complete beginner to the already highly competent musician. So, a word first to the person who plays an instrument well but who now wants to use the instrument for therapeutic exercising. I suggest that you check that your instrument is working the areas of the body which need to be used and possibly consider taking up a different instrument if it does not.

For those who might be thinking of taking up an instrument for the first time, there are several things to take into consideration. What instrument do you enjoy the sound of? What areas of the body do you want to strengthen? What space in your home is available? What can you afford? Could you find a teacher if you want one?

On the question of cost of an instrument, it is always difficult to spend a great deal of money when you don't know whether you will enjoy or be successful at an activity. All instruments come in varying prices, though it's worth remembering that the more you spend, potentially the better the sound produced, which could affect your motivation.

Whether to teach yourself or find a teacher really depends on you. Many people like the support and encouragement of a teacher who can guide their learning specifically where they need it. But this is a self-help book, so I also recommend the many teach yourself books, apps, and piano courses online that Google offers. Or try a combination, teaching yourself until you need specific help, then approach a teacher.

I have taught the piano for 55 years to hundreds of pupils, many of whom have begun as adults. Some have made quick progress, others have taken a steadier pace, but all have reported huge personal satisfaction and enjoyment from learning to produce music. There are various devices on the market for strengthening hands and fingers but exercising with them does not give the pleasure and sense of fulfilment that can come from playing a musical instrument.

Chapter summary

- This chapter has pointed to many ways in which making music can help body, brain and mood:
- Practising slow, deep breathing can reduce stress, depression, pain and fatigue, and help people with COPD, PTSD, IBS, insomnia and speech problems in Parkinson's.
- Singing decreases cortisol and increases endorphin release, oxytocin and boosts immune proteins. It can help anxiety, depression, pain, snoring, sleep apnea, stuttering, and the speech and swallow problems seen in Parkinson's.
- Humming has all the benefits of deep breathing plus benefits for sinuses and increasing nasal nitric oxide.
- Playing an instrument provides physical exercise, enjoyment and personal satisfaction and is an opportunity for self-expression and creativity. It is a complete brain workout involving multiple areas simultaneously, encourages brain plasticity and neurogenesis, and in neurological motor and cognitive problems can activate alternative neural pathways that are not damaged.

Chapter 5

On a personal note...

"Every disease is a musical problem;
every cure is a musical solution"

NOVALIS

It was never my intention to make the focus of this book my personal story. Rather, my aim has been to root the information presented and suggestions made in published research where ideas have been tested on many people. However, several of my friends have insisted that I put in my personal story, saying it was often what interested them most! So, in this final chapter, I will talk of how the power of music has helped and continues to help me on my own Parkinson journey.

Music has been an important part of my life since I was young: singing at school and at church and having piano lessons from the age of seven. During my early teenage years, I played the piano as my school gathered for assembly each morning and later, when in the sixth form, I played the hymns for assembly at a nearby boys' school. Being the only girl surrounded by a few hundred boys was a daunting experience and caused more than the occasional wrong note!

I had always wanted to teach, and when I was considering which college to go to, my piano teacher suggested that I apply to a music college in Manchester. I was surprised at the interview/audition to be offered a place for the next year and very excitedly returned to school to tell my headmaster. As he had heard me playing the hymns at the boys' school, he suggested that I wait till I had their offer in writing before celebrating! But all was well, and I was soon departing for Manchester and music college. Music filled my days and I was very happy. I worked hard, gaining an Associate of the Royal College of Music in piano teaching and winning the piano prize in my second year and graduating from the college at the end of three years.

In the years that followed I taught class music in various schools both in England and in British Forces schools in Germany and Belgium. I also taught piano pupils individually. During this time, I married and had a daughter whom I introduced to music at an early age and who is now a professional flautist.

When I was 50, I heard of a new MA course at Sheffield University, 'Psychology for Musicians'. It brought together two areas of particular interest to me and, as my daughter was by then away from home and I had some free time, I applied and was delighted to be accepted on the course. I enjoyed the topics involved and loved researching and was surprised and rather proud to pass with distinction, the only one in that year. My tutor suggested I consider continuing my studies by doing a PhD, and although I had never considered it was something I could do, I had soon made up my mind to try and four years later I found myself graduating, dressed in cap and gown for the third time.

During this time, I began noticing small motor problems. I found it difficult to double click the mouse to open a file on the computer and my right thumb twitched. Furthermore, the speed at which my right hand could play fast passages on the piano had slowed considerably, something I told myself at the time was probably due to lack of practise. I had an impinged left shoulder, then an impinged right shoulder and I sought the help of a physiotherapist who reassured me that it was probably a trapped nerve and I would soon be able to play the piano as before. But things did not improve, and I decided to ask the opinion of a neurologist.

I did not expect a diagnosis of anything serious and had travelled alone to the appointment. As I described my symptoms, the neurologist looked pleased to tell me I had diagnosed myself very clearly, and that it was Parkinson's. From that moment my future changed. A friend of mine had died of Parkinson's the month before and my grandmother had been an invalid for the last ten years of her life with the disease. I was in shock. Could I be a person with a degenerative brain disorder? Could I be an invalid? It was a part I'd never imagined myself having to play. I returned to my car in tears and tried to phone my husband and my daughter. Neither answered and I drove the one-hour journey home, alone with my thoughts.

Over the next few weeks I deteriorated quickly as I tried on the mantle of Parkinson's. I was frightened and in shock and I was grieving for the life I thought I would no longer be able to lead. Fortunately, my earlier training in research encouraged me to explore the internet for ways in which I could help myself and I was soon exercising and changing my diet.

The piano suffered, however. What was the point in trying to play when I would never be able to play as I used to? What was the point in watching while every week I'd be able to play less and less? In fact, I confess I gave up playing for several years as I grieved for my loss. But in 2016 I heard of a man diagnosed with Parkinson's called Chris Lacey, who had improved his symptoms substantially by spending several hours a day carving chess pieces. (A Google search will offer various newspaper articles on his story). After an email conversation with him, I decided to return to playing the piano, feeling that it would be just as good a therapeutic tool, if not better, than carving chess pieces.

Then in 2017, I met Dr Joaquin Farias, a leading specialist treating dystonia and movement disorders. He is the director of the Neuroplastic Training Institute in Toronto, and he has a background in music. He told me several interesting things, including how walking to music could stimulate an alternative neural pathway in the brain. He whet my appetite to explore the benefits of music for Parkinson's further, which ultimately led to the writing of this book. Dr Farias reinforced my idea that the piano would be a good rehabilitative tool. However, returning to playing the piano was hard for various reasons. First let me attempt to describe how Parkinson's affected my playing and how this differed from simple lack of practice.

From the age of seven till I was 21 I played the piano daily to improve control, speed, technique etc. However, when I started teaching I didn't have the time for daily practice, but the years I had spent playing meant that I could just pick up a piece and play it well enough to cope with the demands of school music teaching. If I was accompanying at a concert, a few hours spent practising the music involved would generally be all that was needed to prepare the music for performance. When Parkinson's affected my playing it did so in different ways and what soon became obvious to me was that a bit of extra practice was not going to make a lot of difference.

Fatigue was one problem. At first I could only play one short piece before the effort of trying to direct and control my fingers had exhausted me and it took six months before I had increased this to three pieces before exhaustion hit. Rigidity, a common problem in Parkinson's, also limited how far my fingers would stretch. And thirdly, my speed of movement was limited. I just couldn't move my hands and fingers fast enough to maintain the rhythm of a tune. These challenges were very different from those which came from lack of practice alone, where one has the energy, flexibility and speed but one lacks the knowledge and kinaesthetic memory of how that particular piece moves across the keyboard.

Yet I have persevered. I have a pile of 20 or 30 music books in which I have flagged over one hundred of my favourite pieces and day by day I work my way through some of them. It is a time in which I am absorbed by the music. If I don't play well one day, I tell myself that it is therapy and therefore it is important *that* I play not *how* I play. Currently I can and do play for an hour each day. I have flexibility back in my fingers and am gradually moving around the keyboard faster. In 2016 I had only hoped to maintain my ability in the face of a degenerative disease but in fact I have improved, dare I say - am still improving. This progress has been very slow and has been more visible by comparing my ability with that of the previous year, rather than comparing progress over months or weeks. It has taken a lot of dogged determination to keep going when my ability was so restricted, not knowing whether I would ever taste again the pleasures of playing a piece well. So why do I think this improvement is happening?

It is not because of any increase in my medication as this, which is still quite a small dose, has stayed the same for five years, which in itself is unusual. When I first read the research discussed and referenced in previous chapters, I realised that the improved ability to play has come about through neuroplasticity and that it's possible that, for movement, my brain could now be using an alternative neural pathway, to take the place of the one which in Parkinson's is not functioning efficiently. Through the amount of practice I have done, I have slowly built a new pathway in my brain to control the movement needed to play the piano, and to control it more efficiently, more effectively and more speedily. I have made demands of my brain with regard to movement and my brain has developed to make my demands possible. Neuroplasticity in action!

I have also noticed other improvements which I believe are a result of my piano playing therapy. My handwriting which was previously slow, is now much quicker and more controlled. I can once more type without finding I have produced countless repeated letters. But I'm hoping playing the piano is giving me further benefits beyond improved strength, flexibility and speed of movement.

In the previous chapter I referred to research which has shown that practising an instrument can produce neuroplasticity in the hippocampus, which is involved in learning and memory. I also suggested that musical practice may boost neurogenesis, the formation of new neurons. I hope that my piano playing is, therefore, also boosting my memory and my thinking. And although I am now in my 70s, I have not noticed any brain fog or memory problems. I still teach and I have written this book, so my cognitive abilities still seem to be in good shape! I am delighted to have the joy of expressing myself through music back in my life and look forward to the time I spend playing the piano each day. But how else do I use music as therapy?

I do listen to music a lot! I have the radio on a music channel most of the day; my preference is usually for classical music. I also play relaxing music during the siesta I take most afternoons. I have made a play list on Spotify, using music I have listed in the appendix, but sometimes I just search 'relaxing piano music' on YouTube. I do find it calms me in times of stress and anxiety.

I have walked to music since Dr Farias first introduced me to its benefits. I relax my shoulders, swing my arms and stride out. Most people would say that I look 'normal' when I walk now. I enjoy stepping in time to my up-beat tracks, which keeps me moving at a good speed and lifts my mood. Although, when I began, I could only manage a walk lasting ten to 15 minutes, I now walk for two and a half miles three-times a week, which takes me about 45 minutes.

During the last few years, my voice and ability to swallow had started to concern me. My friends all reassured me that my voice sounded fine, but I felt it had become lower, with less expression and variation in pitch. I was hardly taking in any breath before I spoke, and my voice sounded and felt tired. It was too much of an effort to sing the hymns in church and, I am embarrassed to say, I gave up. I could not rely on the sound I would make when I began to speak or sing, and I lost a lot of confidence. When inefficient swallowing led to coughing each time I had a drink, I made up my mind that something needed to be done and I began a programme which consisted of ten minutes deep breathing, five minutes humming and 5 to ten minutes singing each day, and after just one month my voice felt stronger and I could hear a big difference in my speaking voice, I can now usually drink a glass of water without coughing and have regained my confidence about being heard in conversations. As I have a slight tendency to be economical with mouth movement and my words are a little slurred at times, I also practise reading to a metronome tick (one syllable per tick) to slow my speech and allow me time to exaggerate mouth and tongue movement. Once again, I have seen improvements quite quickly, the practice encourages better habits and I now generally speak with clearer articulation.

Several years ago, I decided that if I could add or change something that would make me feel just 5% better I would do so because then, after I had found 20 such things, I should feel 100% better. I have kept with this idea and the recommendations in this book represent some of the things which have made me feel better.

I do hope my suggestions for using music to reduce symptoms will be useful to many. If you decide to try one or more of my recommendations, choose a time of day that is usually free and make it a routine to do it at that time. It is always easier to remember to do something if it is a regular commitment at that time. I always walk after breakfast and I play the piano between 5pm and 6pm. If you don't have a regular time, it is easy to forget or to put it off and before you know it the day has gone! I wish you luck with your efforts. What better therapy is there than music, which can stimulate your brain, encourage your body to move, lift your spirits, is safe and inexpensive and can be used alongside other therapies?

Appendices

"Where words fail, music speaks."

HANS CHRISTIAN ANDERSON

Appendix 1

Examples of relaxing music

Classical

- Air on a G string by J S Bach
- Gymnopedie No 1 by Erik Satie
- Shostakovich Piano Concerto no 2, 2nd movement
- 'Romeo and Juliet' by Craig Armstrong
- Chopin Piano Concerto no 1 in E minor 2nd movement
- Spiegel im Spiegel by Arvo Pärt
- 'Ladies in Lavender' by Nigel Hess
- Pie Jesu by John Brunning
- Ave Maria by Schubert
- Double Violin Concerto in D minor, 2nd mov. Largo by J S Bach
- Flute & Harp Concerto K299, 2nd mov. by Mozart
- Piano Concerto K488, no 23, 2nd mov. by Mozart
- Piano Concerto no 2, 2nd mov. by Rachmaninov
- Symphony no 2 in E minor, op 27, 3rd mov. Adagio by Rachmaninov

Easy Listening

- 'Summertime' from Porgy and Bess by George Gershwin
- 'Yesterday' by John Lennon & Paul McCartney
- 'We've only just begun' by Roger Nichols & Paul Williams
- 'Evergreen' by Barbra Streisand & Paul Williams

'New Age', Native American and Indian

- 'Echoes of Time' by C Carlos Nakai from the Canyon Trilogy.
- 'The Winding Path' by Kevin Kern
- Classical Indian Music for healing. 'Peaceful Evening' Raga mix
- 'Native American Earth Drum'
- Buddha Spirit by Aneal and Bradfield

Appendix 2

Examples of sad music

Songs

- Famous Blue Raincoat – Leonard Cohen
- Don't Cry – Guns N' Roses
- Stairway to Heaven – Led Zeppelin
- Still Got the blues – Gary Moore
- Angie – The Rolling Stones
- The River – Bruce Springsteen
- Lovely – Billie Eilish, Khalid
- Dancing With a Stranger – Sam Smith, Normani
- Someone You Loved – Lewis Capaldi
- Lost Without You – Freya Ridings
- Half a Man – Dean Lewis
- Not about angels – Birdy
- When the Party's Over – Billie Eilish

Classical

- Adagio – Samuel Barber
- Miserere – Gregorio Allegri
- Song for Athene – John Tavener
- Hymn to the Fallen – John Williams
- Adagio – Albinoni
- Lacrimosa, Requiem in D minor – Mozart

- Nocturne No 20 in C sharp minor – Chopin
- Schindler's List, main theme – John Williams
- When I am laid in earth (Dido's lament) – Purcell
- Violin Concerto no 1 in G minor, 2nd movement Adagio – Max Bruch

Appendix 3

Examples of music to walk to

The following list of songs is arranged from slow to fast. Decide how fast your step cadence is and then select music for a playlist to use when walking.

Song	Artist	bpm
I Love Rock 'N' Roll	Britney Spears	90
One Shining Moment	Diana Ross	90
Oops! I Did It Again	Britney Spears	95
Overprotected	Britney Spears	96
Lovely Day	Bill Withers	98
I Want You Back	Jackson 5	98
Superstition	Stevie Wonder	99
Crazy In Love	Beyonce	99
Pon De Replay	Rihanna	99
Alejandro	Lady Gaga	99
Suddenly I See	K T Tunstall	100
Unwritten	Natasha Bedingfield	100
Rock Your Body	Justin Timberlake	101
Dancing Queen	Abba	101
Chunky	Bruno Mars	101
Dirty	Christine Aguilera	102
She Will Be Loved	Maroon5	103
Jack And Diane	John Mellencamp	104
Oh What A Night	The Four Seasons	104

Rumour Has It	Adele	120
Teenage Dream	Katy Perry	120
Hummingbird Heartbeat	Katy Perry	120
California Girls	Katy Perry	126

References

*"Music is the language of the spirit.
It opens the secret of life bringing it peace, abol-
ishing strife"*

KAHLIL GIBRAN

Chapter 1: Introduction

Alluri V., Toiviainen P., Jaaskelainen I.P., Glerean E., Sams M., Brattico E. (2011). Large-scale brain networks emerge from dynamic processing of musical timbre, key and rhythm. *Neuroimage.* doi: 10.1016/j. neuroimage.2011.11.019

Ansdell G. (2004). Book review. Music as medicine-The history of music therapy since antiquity. *Psychology of Music,* 32, 440–444

Davison J.T.R. (1899). Music in Medicine. Lancet. 1899:154:1159–62.

Dobrzinska E., Cesarz H., Rymaszewska A. K. (2006). Music therapy - history, definitions and application. *Archives of Psychiatry and Psychotherapy,* 8(1), 47–52

Gfeller, K. E. (2002). Music as a therapeutic agent: Historical and socio-cultural perspectives. *Music therapy in the treatment of adults with mental disorders; theoretical bases and clinical interventions,* 60–67.

Harvey A. W. (1980). The therapeutic role of music in special education; Historical perspectives. *The Creative Child and Adult Quarterly,* 5(3), 196–204.

Stowe R.L., Ives N.J., Clarke C., van Hilton J., Ferreira J., Hawker R.J., Shah L., Wheatley K., Gray R. (2008). Dopamine agonist therapy in early Parkinsons's Disease. *Cochrane Database of Systematic Reviews* 2008, Issue 2. doi: 10.1002/14651858.CD006564.pub2

Chapter 2: Listening to music

Aarsland D., Pahlhagen S., Ballard C.G., Ehrt U., Svenningsson P. (2011). Depression in Parkinson disease: epidemiology, mechanisms and management. *Nat Rev Neurol* 8(1):35–47, doi: 10.1038/nrneurol.2011.189

Angel L.A., Polzella D.J., Elvers G.C. (2010) Background music and cognitive performance. *Percept. Mot. Skills* 11, 1059-1064. doi: 10.2466/pms.1010.3c.1059-1064

Baumgartner T., Esslen M., Jancke L. (2006). From emotion perception to emotion experience: emotions evoked by pictures and classical music. *Int J Psychophysiol* 2006, 60:34-43

Bloor A. (2009). The rhythm's gonna get ya'- background music in primary classrooms and its effect on behavior and attainment. *J. Emot. Behav. Disord.*. 14, 261-274. doi: 10.1080/13632750903303070

Bradt J., Dileo C., Potvin N. (2013) Music for stress and anxiety reduction in coronary heart disease patients. *Cochrane Database of Systematic Reviews* 2013 Issue 12 Art No.:CD006577. doi: 10.1002/14651858.CD006577.pub3

Bringman H., Giesecke K., Thorne A., Bringman S. (2009). Relaxing music as pre-medication before surgery: a randomized con-trolled trial. *Acta Anaesthesiol Scand* 2009 Jul;53(6):759-64. doi: 10.1111/j.1399-6576.2009.01969.x.

Chan M.F., Chan E.A., Mok E., Tse F.Y.K. (2009) Effect of music on depression levels and physiological responses in community-based older adults. *International Journal of Mental Health Nursing*. doi: doi. org/10.1111/j.1447-0349.2009.00614.x

Chan M.F., Chan E.A., Mok E. (2010) Effects of music on depres-sion and sleep quality in elderly people: A randomized controlled trial. *Complementary Therapies in Medicine* 18(3–4):150–159

Chang E.T., Lai H.L., Chen P.W., Hsieh Y.M., Lee L.H. (2012). The effects of music on the sleep quality of adults with chronic insomnia using evidence from polysomnographic and self-reported analysis: a random-ized control trial. *Int J Nurs Stud*. 2012 Aug;49(8):921–30. doi: 10.1016/j. ijnurstu.2012.02.019. Epub 2012 Apr 10.

Cockerton T., Moore S., Norman D. (1997). Cognitive test performance and background music. *Percept Mot Skills* 85, 1435–1438, doi: 10.2466/pms.1997.85.3f.1435

Cortright B. (2015). *The Neurogenesis diet and lifestyle, upgrade your brain, upgrade your life.* Psychic Media

Esfandiari D., Mansouri S. (2014) The effect of listening to light and heavy music on reducing the symptoms of depression among female students. *The Arts in Psychotherapy.* 41(2):211-213. doi: doi.org/10.1016/j.aip.2014.02.001

Fallek R., Corey K., Qamar A., Vernisie S.N., Hoberman A., Selwyn P.A., Fausto J.A., Marcus P., Kvetan V., Lounsbury D.W.(2019). Soothing the heart with music: A feasibility study of bedside music therapy intervention for critically ill patients in an urban hospital setting. *Palliative Support Care* doi: doi.org/10.1017/S147895159000294.

Ferreri l., Aucouturier J.J., Muthalib M.,Bigand E., Bugaiska A. (2013). Music improves verbal memory encoding while decreasing prefrontal cortex activity: an fNIRS study. *Front Hum Neuroscience,* 7:779, doi: 10.3389/fnhum.2013.00779.

Ford B. (2010). Pain in Parkinson's disease. *Mov Disord* 2010;25 Suppl 1:S 98-103. doi: 10.1002/mds.22716

Furnham A., Bradley A. (1997). Music while you work: the differential distraction of background music on the cognitive test performance of introverts and extroverts. *Appl. Cogn. Psychol.* 11, 445-455. doi: 10.1002/(sici)1099-0720(199710)11:5<445::aid-acp472>3.3.co;2-i

Gabrielsson A., Lindstrom E (2010). The role of structure in the musical expression of emotion. In Juslin P.N., Sloboda J.A. (Eds), *Handbook of music and emotion: Theory, research, applications.* Oxford University Press. 367–400

Garrido S., Schubert E. (2013) Moody melodies: Do they cheer us up? A study of the effect of sad music on mood. *Psychology of Music.* doi: doi.org/10.1177/0305735613501938

Garza-Villarreal E.A., Wilson A.D., Vase L., Brattico E., Barrios F.A., Jensen T.S., Romero-Romo J.I., Vuust P. (2014) Music reduces pain and increases functional mobility in fibromyalgia. *Frontiers in Psychology.* doi; 10.3389/f.psyg.2014.00090

Gjerstad, M.D., Wentzel-Larsen T., Larsen J.P. (2007). Insomnia in Parkinson's disease: frequency and progression over time. *J Neurol Neurosurg Psychiatry.* 2007 May:78(5);476–479

Gold A., Clare A. (2012). An exploration of music listening in chronic pain. *Psychology of Music* doi.org/10.1177/0305735612440613

Hallam S., Price J. (1998). Research section: can the use of background music improve the behavior and academic performance of children with emotional and behavioral difficulties? *Br. J. Spec. Educ.* 25, 88-91. doi: 10.1111/1467–8527.t01-1-00063

Harmat L., Takacs J., Bodizs R (2008). Music improves sleep quality in students. *J Adv Nurs.* 2008 May;62(3):327-35 doi: 10.1111/j.1365-2648.2008.04602.x.

Hsu C-C., Chen S-R., Lee P-H. (2017). The effect of music listening on pain, heart rate variability, and range of motion in older adults after total knee replacement. *Clinical Nursing Research* doi.org/10.1177/1054773817749108

Husain G., Thompson W.F., Shellenberg E.G. (2002). Effects of musical tempo and mode on arousal, mood and spatial abilities. *Music Percept.* 20, 151–171. doi: 10.1525/mp.2002.20.2.151

Jancke L. (2008). Music, memory and emotion. *Journal of Biology.* 2008, 7:21. doi: 10.1186/jbiol82

Jhaveri D.J., Tedoldi A., Hunt S., Sullivvan R., Watts N.R., Power J.M., Bartlett P.F., Sah P. (2018). Evidence for newly generated interneurons in the basolateral amygdala of adult mice. *Molecular Pscyhiatry* 23: 521–532

Kampfe J., Sedlmeier P., Renkewitz F. (2010). The impact of background music on adult listeners: a meta-analysis. *Psychol. Music* 39,424–448. doi: 10.1177/0305735610376261

Kane E., (1914) The phonograph in the operating room. *JAMA* 1914;62;1829-30.

Kang H.L., Williamson J.W. (2013). Background music can aid second language learning. *Psychol Music* 42, 728-747, doi: 10.1177/0305735613485152

Khalfa S., Dalla Bella S., Roy M., Peretz I., Lupien S.J. (2003). Effects of relaxing music on Salivary Cortisol level after Psychological Stress. *Ann N Y Acad Sci* 2003 Nov;999:374–6

Kim H., Lee M-H., Chang H-K., Lee T-H., Lee H-H., Shin M-C., Shin M-S., Won R., Shin H-S., Kim C-J. (2006). Influence of prenatal noise and music on the spatial memory and neurogenesis in the hippocampus of developing rats. *Brain & Development.* (2006) 109–114.

Kim C-H., Lee S-C., Shin J.W., Chung K-J., Lee S-H., Shin M-S., Baek S-B., Sung Y-H., Kim C-J., Kim K-H. (2013). Exposure to Music and Noise During Pregnancy Influences Neurogenesis and Thickness in Motor and Somatosensory Cortex of Rat Pups. *Int. Neurourol J.* 2013;17:107–113. doi: dxx.doi.org/10.5213/inj.2013.17.3.107

Koelsch S., Fuermetz J., Sack U., Bauer K., Hohenadel M., Wiegel M., Kaisers U.X., Heinke W. (2011). Effects of music listening on cortisol levels and propofol consumption during spinal anesthesia. *Frontiers in Psychology.* 2011 doi:10.3389/fpsyg 2011.00058

Lai H. L., Good M. (2005). Music improves sleep quality in older adults. *J Adv Nurs.* 2005 Feb;49(3):234–244

Lee O.K.A., Chung Y.F.L., Chan M.F., Chan W.M. (2005). Music and its effect on the physiological responses and anxiety levels of patients receiving mechanical ventilation; a pilot study. *Journal of Clinical Nursing* (2005) doi: doi.org/10.1111/j.1365-2702.2004.01103.x.

Marzban M., Shabbatzi A., Tondar M., Soleimani M., Bakhshayesh M., Moshkforoush A., Sadati M., Zendehrood S.A., Joghayaei M.T. (2011). Effect of Mozart music on hippocampal content of BDNF in postnatal rats. *Basic and Clinical Neuroscience.* Spring 2011: 2(3)

Millgram Y., Joorman J., Huppert J.D., Tamir M. (2015) Sad as a matter of choice? Emotion-regulation goals in depression. *Psychological Science*, 26, 1216-1228 doi: doi.org/10.1177/0956797615583295

Miskovic D., Rosenthal R., Zingg U., Oertli D., Metzger U., Jancke L. (2008). Randomized controlled trial investigating the effect of music on the virtual reality laparoscopic learning performance of novice surgeons. *Surg. Endosc.* 22, 2416–2420. doi: 10.1007/s00464-008-0040-8

Mizuno T., Sugishita M. (2007). Neural correlates underlying perception of tonality-related emotional contents. *Neuroreport* 2007, 18:1651–1655

Oliver M. (1997). The effect of background music on mood and reading comprehension performance of at-risk college freshman. *Dissertation Abstr.* 57, 5039

Peretz I., Corbeil M., Trehub S. (2015). Singing delays the onset of infant distress. *Infancy.* Published online 22 Sept.2015. doi: 10.1111/infa.12114

Pimenta M., Moreira D., Nogueira T., Silva C., Pinto E.B., Valenca G.T., Ameida L.R.S. (2018). Anxiety independently contributes to severity of freezing of gait in people with Parkinson Disease. *The Journal of Neuropsychiatry and Clinical Neurosciences.* Published online:6 Sept 2018 doi.org/10.1176/appi.neuropsych

Rana A.Q., Qureshi A.R.M., Haris A., Danish M.A., Furqan M.S., Shaikh O. (2018). Negative impact of severity of pain on mood, social life and general activity in Parkinson's disease. *Neurological Research* Pages 1054-1059 doi.org/10.1080/01616412.2018.1517852

Rauscher F.H., Shaw G.L., Ky K.N. (1993) Music and spatial task performance. *Nature* 365, 611.

Routh L.C., Black J.L., Ahlskog J.E., (1987). Parkinson's Disease complicated by anxiety. *Mayo Clin Proc* 1987, 62:733–735

Sarkamo T., Tervaniemi M., Laicinen S.,Forsblom A, Soinila S., Mikkonen M.,Autti T., Silvennoinen H.M., Erkkila J., Laine M., Peretz I., Hietanen M. (2008). Music listening enhances cognitive recovery and mood after middle cerebral artery stroke. *Brain.* 2006, 131:866-876.

Seritan A.L., Rienas C., Duong T., Delucchi K., Ostrem J.L. (2019). Ages at Onset of Anxiety and Depressive Disorders in Parkinson's Disease. *The Journal of Neuropsychiatry and Clinical Neurosciences.* Published online:23 May 2019

Shifriss R., Bodner E., Palgi Y. (2014) When you're down and troubled. Views on the regulatory power of music. *Psychology of Music.* doi: doi. org/10.1177/0305735614540360

Siedlieck S.L., Good M. (2006). Effect of music on power, pain, depression and disability. *Journal Advanced Nursing.* Jun;54(5):553–62 doi: 10.1111/j.1365-2648.2006.03860.x.

Simavli S., Gumus I., Kaygusuz I., Yildirim M., Usluogullari B., Kafali H. (2014). Effect of music on labor pain relief, anxiety level and postpartum analgesic requirement: A randomized controlled clinical trial. *Gynecologic and Obstetric Investigation.* 2014;78:244–250 doi.org/10.1159/000365085

Starkstein S.E., Preziosi T.J., Bolduc P.L., Robinson R.G. (1990). Depression in Parkinson's disease. *Journal of Nervous and Mental Disease* 178(1):27–31

Su C.P., Lai H.L., Chang E. T.,Yiin L.M., Perng S.J.,Chen P.,W. (2013). A randomized controlled trial of the effects of listening to non-commercial music on quality of nocturnal sleep and relation indices in patients in medical intensive care unit. *J.Adv Nurs* 2013 Jun;69(6):1377–89. doi: 10.1111/j.1365-2648.2012.06130.x. Epub 2012 Aug 29

Thompson W.F., Schellenberg E.G., Husain G. (2001). Arousal, mood and the Mozart effect. *Psychol. Sci.* 12, 248–251. doi: 10.1111/1467-9280.00345

Van den Tol A.J.M., Edwards J., Heflick N.A., (2016). Sad music as a means for acceptance-based coping. *Musicae Scientiae.* doi: doi. org/10.1177/1029864915627844

Van Hilton B., Hoff J.I., Middelkoop H.A., van der Velde E.A., Kerkhof G.A., Wauquire A., Kamphuisen H.A., Roos R.A. (1994). Sleep disruption in Parkinson's disease. Assessment by continuous activity monitoring. *Arch Neurol* 199451922–928.

Voss J.A., Good M., Yates B., Baun M.M., Thompson A., Hertzog M.A. (2004). Sedative music reduces anxiety and pain during chair rest after open-heart surgery. *Pain.* doi: 10.1016/j.pain.2004.08.020

Walsh K., Bennett G., (2001). Parkinson's disease and anxiety. *Postgrad Med J*, 77; 89–93

Wang C. F., Sun Y.L., Zang H.X. (2014). Music therapy improves sleep quality in acute and chronic sleep disorders: a meta-analysis of 10 randomized studies. *Int J Nurs Stud* 2014 Jan;51(1):51-62. doi: 10.1016/j. ijnurstu.2013.03.008. Epub 2013 Apr 9.

Watchi M. Koyama M., Utsuyama M., Bittman B.B., Kiagawa M., Hirokawa K. (2007). Recreational music making modulates natural killer cell activity, cytokines and mood states in corporate employees. *Med Sci Monit* 2007;13:CR57-70

Weth K., Raab M.H., Carbon C-C. (2015) Investigating emotional responses to self-selected sad music via self-report and automated facial analysis. *Musicae Scientiae* doi: doi.org/10.1177/1029864915606796

Yoon S., Verona E., Schlauch R., Schneider S., Rottenberg J. (2019) Why do depressed people prefer sad music? *Emotion* doi: dx.doi.org/10.1037/ emo0000573

Chapter 3: Moving to Music

Ahlskog J.E. (2011). Does vigorous exercise have a neuroprotective effect in Parkinson's disease? *Neurology* 77:288–294.

Allen J.L., McKay J.L., Sawers A., Hackney M.E., Ting L.H. (2017). Increased neuromuscular consistency in gait and balance after part-nered, dance-based rehabilitation in Parkinson's disease. *Journal of Neurophysiology.* 2017, Jul 1;118(1)363–373. doi: 10.1152/jn.00813.2016

Arias P., Cudeiro J. (2008). Effects of rhythmic sensory stimulation (audi-tory, visual) on gait in Parkinson's disease patients. *Exp Brain Res.* 2008 Apr;186(4)589-601. doi: 10.1007/s00221-007-1263-y.

Baker K., Rochester L., Nieuwboer A. (2008). The effect of cues on gait variability, Reducing the attentional cost of walking in people with Parkinson's disease. *Parkinsonism and Related Disorders* 14(4); 314–320. doi. org/10.1016/j.parkreldis.2007.09.008

Baram Y., Miller A. (2007). Auditory feedback control for improvement of gait in patients with Multiple Sclerosis. *J. Neurol. Sci.* Mar 15;254(1–2):90-4 doi: 10.1016/j.jns.2007.01.003

Baram Y., Lenger R. (2011). Gait improvement in patients with cere-bral palsy by visual and auditory feedback. *Neuromodulation* 2012 Jan-Feb;15(1):48–52.. doi: 10.1111/j.1525-1403.2011.00412.x.

Bayod S., del Valle J., Canudas A.M., Lalanza J.F., Sanchez-Roige S., Camins A., Escorihuela R.M., Pallas M. (2011). Long-term treadmill exer-cise induces neuroprotective molecular changes in rat brain. *J. Appl. Physiol.* 111: 1380–1390, 2011. doi: 10.1152/applphysiol.00425.2011.

Bill J.M. (1967). Demonstration of the traditional approach in the treat-ment of a patient with parkinsonism. *American Journal of Physical Medicine.* 46, 1034–1036

Blin O., Ferrandez A.M., Serratrice G. (1990). Quantitative analysis of gait in Parkinson patients; increased variability of stride length. *J.Neurol.Sci.* 98,91–97. doi: 10.1016/0022-510X(90)90184-O

Bradt J., Magee W.L., Dileo C., Wheeler B.L., McGilloway E. (2010). Music therapy for acquired brain injury. *Cochrane Database Syst Rev.* 2010 Jul 7;(7):CD006787. doi:10.1002/14651858.CD006787.pub2.

Brown L.A., de Bruin N., Doan J.B., Suchowersky O., Hu B. (2009). Novel challenges to gait in Parkinson's disease: the effect of concurrent music in single- and dual- task contexts. *Arch. Phys. Med Rehabil.* 2009 Sep;90(9):1578–83. doi: 10.1016/j.apmr.2009.03.009.

Brown L.A., de Bruin N., Doan J.B., Suchowersky O., Hu B.(2010). Obstacle crossing among people with Parkinson disease is influenced by concurrent music. *Journal of Rehabilitation, Research and Development.* 47(3): 225–232.

Buard I., Teale P., Rojas D.C., Kronberg E., Thaut M.H., Kluger B.M., Dewispelaere W.B. (2019). Auditory entrainment of motor responses in older adults with and without Parkinson's disease: an MEG study. *Neuroscience Letters* 2019 Jun 18,708:134331

Conklyn D., Stough D., Novak E., Paczak S., Chemali K., Bethoux F. (2010). A home-based walking program using rhythmic auditory stimulation improves gait performance in patients with multiple sclerosis: a pilot study. *Neurorehabil Neural Repair.* 2010 Nov-Dec:24(9):835–842. doi: 10.1177/1545968310372139

Costas M.B., Karageorghis I., Hoy G.K., Layne G.S. (2019). The way you make me feel: Psychological and cerebral responses to music during real-life physical activity. *Psychology of Sport and Exercise* Vol 41, March 2019, Pages 211–217. doi: doi.org/10.1016/j.psychsport.2018.01.010

Debaere F., Wenderoth N., Sunaert S., Van Hecke P., Swinnen S.P. (2003). Internal vs external generation of movements: differential neural pathways involved in bimanual coordination performed in the presence of absence of augmented visual feedback. *Neurolmage* 19, 763–776.

De Bruin N., Doan J.B., Turnbull G., Suchowersky O., Bonfield S., Hu B., Brown L.A. (2010). Walking with Music is a safe and viable tool for gait training inn Parkinson's Disease: The effect of a 13-week feasibility study on single and dual task walking. *Parkinson's Disease*. Vol 2010, Article ID 483530, 9 pages. doi: 10.4061/2010/483530.

Ebersbach G., Heijmenberg M., Kindermann L., Trottenberg T., Wissel J., Poewe W. (1999). Interference of rhythmic constraint on gait in healthy subjects and patients with early Parkinson's disease; evidence for impaired locomotor pattern generation in early Parkinson's disease. *Movement Disorders: Official Journal of the Movement Disorder Society* 14, 619–625.

Farley B.G., Fox C.M., Ramig L.O., McFarland D.H. (2008). Intensive amplitude-specific therapeutic approaches for Parkinson's disease. *Topics in Geriatric Rehabilitation* Vol. 24, No, 2, pp. 99–114

Fernández-del-Olmo M., Cudeiro J. (2003). A simple procedure using auditory stimuli to improve movement in Parkinson's disease: a pilot study. *Neurology & Clinical Neurophysiology*, 1–7.

Hackney M.E., Earhart G.M. (2009). Effects of dance on gait and balance in Parkinson's disease: A comparison of partnered and non-partnered dance movement. *Neurorehabilitation and neurol repair*. doi.org/10.1177/1545968309353329

Hackney M.E., Earhart G.M. (2010). Effects of dance on balance and gait in severe Parkinson disease: A case study. *Disability and rehabilitation*. 2010;32(8(:679-84. doi: 10.3109/096382800903247905

Hausdorff J.M., Lowenthal J., Herman T., Gruendlinger L., Peretz C., Giladi N. (2007). Rhythmic auditory stimulation modulates gait variability in Parkinson's disease. *Eur J Neurosci*. 2007 Oct,26(8):2369–2375. doi 10.1111/j.1460-9568.2007.05810.x.

Howe T.E., Lovegreen B., Cody F.W., Ashton V.J., Oldham J.A. (2003). Auditory cues can modify the gait of persons with early-stage Parkinson's disease: a method for enhancing parkinsonian walking performance? *Clin. Rhabil.* 2003 Jul;17(4):363–367. doi: 10.1191/0269215503cr621oa.

Hurt C.P., Rice R.R., McIntosh G.C., Thaut M.H. (1998). Rhythmic Auditory Stimulation in Gait Training for Patients with Traumatic Brain Injury. *J. Music Ther.* 1998;35(4):228–241

Jankovic J. (2015). Gait disorders. *Neurol Clin* (2015). 33(1):249–68 doi: 10.1016/j.ncl.2014.09.007

Jones C.R., Malone T.J., Dirnberger G., Edwards M., Jahanshahi M. (2008). Basal ganglia, dopamine and temporal processing; performance on three timing tasks on and off medication in Parkinson's Disease. *Brain and Cognition* 68, 30–41.

Kadivar Z., Corcos D.M., Foto J., Hondzinski J.M. (2011). Effect of step training and rhythmic auditory stimulation on functional performance in Parkinson patients. *Neurorehabil Neural Repair.* 2011 Sept;25(7):626–635. doi: 10.1177/1545968311401627.

Kim S.J., Kwak E.E., Park E.S., Cho S.R. (2012). Differential effects of rhythmic auditory stimulation and neurodevelopmental treatment/Bobath on gait patterns in adults with cerebral palsy: a randomized controlled trial. *Clin. Rehabil.* 2012 Oct;26(10):904–914. doi: 10.1177/0269215511434648.

Kleim J.A., Cooper N.R. Vandenberg P.M. (2002). Exercise induces angiogenesis but does not alter movement representations within rat motor cortex. *Brain Research* 934, 1–6

Kwak E.E. (2007). Effect of rhythmic auditory stimulation on gait performance in children with spastic cerebral palsy. *J. Music Ther.* 2007 Fall;44(3):198–216

Lim H.A., Miller K., Fabian C. (2011). The effects of therapeutic instrumental music performance on endurance level, self-perceived fatigue level and self-perceived exertion of inpatients in physical rehabilitation. *J Music The.* 2011;48(2):124–48

McIntosh G.C., Brown S.H., Rice R.R., Thaut M.H. (1997). Rhythmic auditory-motor facilitation of gait patterns in patients with Parkinson's disease. *Journal of Neurology, Neurosurgery and Psychiatry.* 1997;62:22-26. doi: 10.1136/jnnp.62.1.22

Miller R.A., Thaut M.H., McIntosh G.C., Rice R.R. (1996). Components of EMG symmetry and variability in Parkinsonian and healthy elderly gait. *Electroencephalography and Clinical Neurophysiology,* 101, 1–7

Moumdjian L., Buhmann J., Willems I., Feys P., Leman M. (2018). Entrainment and synchronization to auditory stimuli during walking in healthy and neurological populations: a methodological systematic review. *Frontiers in Human Neuroscience* June 2018, Vol 12, Article 263. doi: 10.3389/fnhum.2018.00263

O'Sullivan S.B., Schmitz T.J. (2007). *Physical Rehabilitation*, 5th edition. Philadelphia, PA: F.A. Davis Company.

Satoh M., Kuzuhara S. (2008). Training in mental singing while walking improves gait disturbance in Parkinson's disease patients. *Eur Neurol.* 2008; 60(5):237–243: doi: 10.1159/000151699.

Tajiri N., Yasuhara T., Shingo T., Kondo A., Yuan W.,Kadota T., Wang F., Baba T., Tayra J. T., Morimoto T., Jing M., Kikuchi Y., Kuramoto S., Agari T., Miyoshi Y.,Fujino H., Obata F., Takeda I., Date I. (2009). Exercise exerts neuroprotective effects on Parkinson's disease model of rats. *J. Brain Res.* doi: doi.org/10.1016/j.brainres.2009.10.075

Thaut C.P., and Rice R. (2014). Rhythmic auditory stimulation (RAS). In Thaut M.H., Hoemberg V. (Eds) (2014) *Handbook of Neurologic Music Therapy.* Oxford University Press. 94–105.

Thaut, M.H., McIntosh G.C., Rice R.R., Miller R.A., Rathbun J., Brault J.M. (1996) Rhythmic auditory stimulation in gait training for Parkinson's disease patients. *Movement Disorders*, 11, 193–200.

Thaut M.H., Kenyon G.P., Schauer M.L., McIntosh G.C. (1999). The connection between rhythmicity and brain function. *IEEE Engineering in Medicine and Biology Magazine; the Quarterly Magazine of the Engineering in Medicine & Biology Society* 18, 101–108.

Van Praag H., Shubert T., Zhao C., Gage F.H. (2005). Exercise enhances learning and hippocampal neurogenesis in aged mice. *The Journal of Neuroscience* 25(38):8680–8685

Von Wilzenben H.D. (1942). *Methods in the Treatment of Postencephalic Parkinson's*. New York: Grune and Stratten.

Willems A.M., Nieuwboer A., Chavret F., Desloovere K., Dom R., Rochester L., Kwakkel G., van Wegen E., Jones D. (2007). Turning in Parkinson's disease patients and controls: the effect of auditory cues. *Move Disord.* 2007 Oct 15;22(13):1871–1878

Chapter 4: Making music

Allen N.E., Canning C.G., Sherrington C., Fung V.S. (2009). Bradykinesia, muscle weakness and reduced muscle power in Parkinson's disease. *Mov Disord* 2009; 24: 1344–1351

Andrews G., Howie P.M., Dozsa M., Guitar B.E. (1982). Stuttering: Speech pattern characteristic under fluency-inducing conditions. *Journal of Speech and Hearing Research.* 1982; 25: 208–216

Baille G., Perez T., Devos D., Deken V., Defebvre L., Moreau C. (2018). Early occurrence of inspiratory muscle weakness in Parkinson's disease. *Journal PLoS One* doi.org/10.1371/journal.pone.019400

Bengtsson S.L., Nagy Z., Forsman L., Forssberg H., Ullen F. (2005). Extensive piano practicing has regionally specific effects on white matter development. *Nat Neurosci.* 2005; 8(9): 1148–1150. doi: 10.1038/nn1516.

Brendel B., Ziegler W. (2008). Effectiveness of metrical pacing in the treatment of apraxia of speech. *Aphasiology*, 22, 77–102

Bunton K. (2005). Patterns of lung volume use during an extemporaneous speech task in persons with Parkinson disease. *Journal of Communication Disorders*. 2005;38:331–348.

Busch V., Magarl W., Kern U., Haas J., Hajak G., Eichhammer P. (2012). The effect of deep and slow breathing on pain perception, autonomic activity and mood processing – An experimental study. *Pain Medicine* 2012; 13: 215–228

Chodzinski J. (2000). The effect of rhythmic breathing on blood pressure in hypertensive adults. *J Undergrad Res.* 2000:1(6)

Chung L-J., Tsai P-S., Liu B-Y., Chou K-R., Lin W-H, Shyu Y-K., Wang M-Y. (2010). Home-based deep breathing for depression in patients with coronary heart disease: A randomised controlled trial. *International Journal of Nursing Studies.* 47(11): 1346–1353. doi:org/10.1016/j.ijnurstu.2010.03.007

Clift S.M., Hancox G. (2001). The perceived benefits of singing: findings from preliminary surveys of a university college choral society. *J R Soc Promot Health* 2001; 121(4):248–256

Clift S., Hancox G., Morrison I., Hess B., Kreutz G., Stewart D. (2010). Choral singing and psychological wellbeing: quantitative and qualitative findings from English choirs in a cross-national survey. *Journal of Applied Arts and Health.* 1(1): 19–34. doi: 10.1386/jaah.1.1.19/1

Cohen G D., Perlstein S., Chapline J., Kelly J., Firth K M., Simmens S. (2006). The impact of professionally conducted cultural programs on the physical health, mental health and social functioning of older adults. *The Gerontologist.* 46(6): 726–734.

Consolo K., Fusner S., Staib S. (2008). Effects of diaphragmatic breathing on stress levels of nursing students. *Teaching and Learning in Nursing.* 3(2): 67–71 doi.org/10.1016/j.teln.2007.10.003

Cooper S., Oborne J., Newton S., Harrison V., Thompson Coon J., Lewis S., Tattersfield A. (2003). Effect of two breathing techniques (Buteyko and pranayama) in asthma: a randomized controlled trial. *Thorax* 2003;58(8):674–679

Darley F.L., Aronson A.E., Brown J.R. (1969). Differential diagnostic patterns of dysarthria. *J Speech Hear Res* 1969,12:246–269

Daykin N., Mansfield L., Meads C., Julier G., Tomlinson A., Payne A., Grigsby Duffy L., Lane J., D'Innocenzo G., Burnett A., Kay T., Dolan P., Testoni S., Victor C. (2017). What works for wellbeing? A systematic review of wellbeing outcomes for music and signing in adults. *Perspectives in public health.* doi.org/10.1177/1757913917740391

Dunbar R.I.M., Kaskatis K., MacDonald I., Barra V. (2012). Performance of music elevates pain threshold and positive affect: implications for the evolutionary function of music. *Evolutionary Psychology.* 2012; 10(4): 688–702

Eby G.A. (2006). Strong humming for one hour daily to terminate chronic rhinosinusitis in four days: a case report and hypothesis for action by stimulation of endogenous nasal nitric oxide production. *Med Hypotheses* 2006; 66(4): 851–4

Elefant C., Baker F.A., Lotan M., Lagesen S.K., Skeie G.O. (2012). The effect of group music therapy on mood, speech and singing in individuals with Parkinson's disease – a feasibility study. *J Music Ther.* 2012; 49(3): 278–302

Fancourt D., Williamon A., Carvalho L A., Steptoe A., Dow R., Lewis I. (2016). Singing modulates mood, stress, cortisol, cytokine and neuropeptide activity in cancer patients and carers. *Ecancermedicalscience*, 2016; 10 doi: 10.3332/ecancer.2016.631

Fancourt D., Perkins R. (2018). Effect of singing interventions on symptoms of postnatal depression: three-arm randomized controlled trial. *The British Journal of Psychiatry.* 212(2): 119–121. doi: doi.org/10.1192/bjp.2017.29

Fernandes M., Cukier A., Feltrim M.I.Z. (2011). Efficacy of diaphragmatic breathing in patients with chronic obstructive pulmonary disease. *Chronic Respiratory Disease.* 8(4):237–244. doi: 10.1177/1479972311424296

Fisher B., Petzinger G., Nixon K. Hogg E., Bremmer S., Meshul C.K., Jacowec M.W. (2004). Exercise induced behavioral recovery and neuroplasticity in the 1-methyl-4-phenyl-1,2,3,6-tetrahydropyridine-lesioned basal ganglia. *J Neurosci Res.* 2004; 77: 378–390

Flasskamp A., Kotz S.A., Schlegel U., Skodda S. (2012). Acceleration of syllable repetition in Parkinson's disease is more prominent in the left-side dominant patients. *Parkinsonism and Related Disorders*;18.343–347

Fogg-Rogers L., Buetow S., Talmage A., McCann C.M., Leao S H.S., Tippett L. (2015). Choral singing therapy following stroke or Parkinson's disease: an exploration of participants' experiences. *Disability and Rehabilitation.* doi: doi.org/10.3109/09638288.2015.1068875

Francois C., Grau-Sanchez J., Duarte E., Rodriguez-Fornells A. (2015). Musical training as an alternative and effective method for neuro-education and neuro-rehabilitation. *Frontiers in Psychology.* doi: 10.3389/fpsyg.2015.00475.

Gaser C, Schlaug G. (2003). Brain structures differ between musicians and non-musicians. *Journal of Neuroscience.* 2003; 23: 9240–9245

Glover H., Kalinowski J., Rastatter M, Stuart A. (1996). Effect of instruction to sing on stuttering frequency at normal and fast rates. *Percept Mot Skills.* doi: doi.org/10.2466/pms.1996.83.2.511

Haneishi E. (2001). Effects of a music therapy voice protocol on speech intelligibility, vocal acoustic measures and mood of individuals with Parkinson's disease. *Journal of Music Therapy.* 2001; 38:273–290

Hartelius L., Svensson P. (1994). Speech and swallowing symptoms associated with Parkinson's disease and Multiple Sclerosis: a survey. *Folia Phoniatrica et Logopaedica.* 1994;46:9-17. doi.org/10/1159/000266286

Healey E.C., Mallard A.R., Adams M.R. (1976). Factors contributing to the reduction of stuttering during singing. *Journal of Speech and Hearing Research.* 1976; 19: 475–480

Higgins A.N., Richardson K.C. (2019). The effects of choral singing intervention on speech characteristics in individuals with Parkinson's disease: an exploratory study. *Communications disorders quarterly.* 2019; 40(4). doi: doi. org/10.1177/1525740118783040

Hilton M.P., Savage J., Hunter B., McDonald S., Repanos C., Powell R. (2013). Singing exercises improve sleepiness and frequency of snoring among snorers – A randomized controlled trial. *International Journal of Otolaryngology and Head and Neck Surgery.* 2013, 2, 97–102. doi: dx.doi. org/10.4236/ijohns.2013.23023

Houston D.M., McKee K.J., Carroll L., Marsh H. (1998). Using humour to promote psychological wellbeing in residential homes for older people. *Aging and Mental Health*, 2(4): 328–332

Hyde K.L., Lerch J., Norton A., Forgeard M., Winner E., Evans A.C., Schlaug G. (2009). Musical training shapes structural brain development. *J Neurosci* 2009; 29(10): 3019–3025. doi: 10.1523/ JNEUROSCI.5118-08.2009

Ingham R J., Bothe A.K., Jang E., Yates L., Cotton J., Seybol I. (2009). Measurement of speech effort during fluency-inducing conditions in adults who do and do not stutter. *Journal of Speech, Language and Hearing Research.*, 52, 1286–1301

Irons J., Hancox G., Stewart D. (2019). Sing to beat Parkinson's: A group singing intervention for people with Parkinson's and their carers. *Mov Disord* 2018; 33(2).

Jerath R., Edry J.W., Barnes V.A., Jerath V. (2006). Physiology of long pranayama breathing: Neural respiratory elements may provide a mechanism that explains how slow deep breathing shifts the autonomic nervous system. *Medical Hypotheses.* 67(3): 566–571.

Judd M., Pooley A. (2013). The psychological benefits of participating in group singing for members of the general public. *Psychology of Music*. doi. org/10.1177/0305735612471237

Kalyani B.G., Venkatasubramanian G., Arasappa R., Rao N.P., Kalmady S.V., Beher R.V., Rao H., Vasudev M.K., Gangadhar B N. (2011). Neurohemodynamic correlates of 'OM' chanting: A pilot functional magnetic resonance imaging study. *International Journal of Yoga* 2011; 4(1): 3–6

Karlsen K.H., Tandberg E., Arsland D., Larsen J. (2000). Health related quality of life in Parkinson's disease: a prospective longitudinal study. *J. Neurol Neurosurg Psychiatr*. 69:584–589

Keeler J.R., Roth E.A., Neuser B.L., Spitsbergen J.M., Waters D.J.M., Viannay J-M. (2015). The neurochemistry and social flow of singing: bonding and oxytocin. *Frontiers in Human Neuroscience*. doi:10.3389/fnhum.2015.00518

Kim S.H., Schneider S.M., Kravitz L., Mermier C., Burge M.R. (2013). Mind-body practices for Post-Traumatic Stress Disorder. *J Investig Med*. 2013:61(5):827–834. doi: 10.231/ jim.0b013e3182906862

Kolbe B., Mohammod A. (2014). Harnessing the power of neuroplasticity for intervention. *Front Hum Neurosci* 8: 377. doi:10.3389/fnhum.2014.00377

Krampe R.T., Ericsson K.A. (1996). Maintaining excellence: deliberate practice and elite performance in young and older pianists. *J Exp Psychol Gen*. 125: 331–359. doi: 10.1037/0096-3445.125.4.331

Kreutz G., Bongard S., Rohmann S., Hodapp V., Grebe D. (2004). Effects of choir singing or listening on secretory immunoglobin A, cortisol and emotional state. *J Behav Med*. 2004; 27(6):623–635

Lakhan S.E., Schofield K.L. (2013). Mindfulness-based therapies in the treatment of somatization disorders: a systematic review and meta-analysis. *Journal PLoS One*. doi.org/10.1371/journal.pone.0071834

Langmore S.E., Pisegna J.M. (2015). Efficacy of exercises to rehabilitate dysphagia: A critique of the literature. *International Journal of Speech-Language Pathology.* doi: 10.3109/17549507.2015.1024171

Lee M.A., Prentice W.M., Hildreth A.J., Walker R.W. (2007). Measuring symptom load in idiopathic Parkinson's disease. *Parkinsonism Relat Disord.* 16(7):284–289

Ludlow C.L. (2005). Central nervous system control of the laryngeal muscles in humans. *Respir Physiol Neurobiol* 2005; 147(2-3): 205–222. doi: 10.1016/j.resp.2005.04.015

Mainka, S. and Mallien, G. (2014). Rhythmic Speech Cueing (RSC). In Thaut M.H. and Hoemberg V. (Eds) *Handbook of Neurologic Music Therapy.* Oxford University Press, 150–160

Martarelli D., Cocchioni M., Scuri S., Pompei P. (2011). Diaphragmatic breathing reduces exercise-induced oxidative stress. *Evidence-based Complementary and Alternative Medicine* Vol 2011 Article ID 932430. doi. org/10.1093/ecam/nep169.

Mateos-Toset S., Cabrera-Martos I., Torres-Sanchez I., Ortiz-Rubio A., Gonzalez-Jimenez E., Valenza M.C. (2015). Effects of a single hand-exercise session on manual dexterity and strength in persons with Parkinson disease: A randomized controlled trial. *J Phy Med Rehabil.* doi: dx.doi.org/10.1016/j. pmrj.2015.06.004

Matthews R., Purdy S., Tippett L. (2018). Acoustic, respiratory, cognitive and wellbeing comparisons of two groups of people with Parkinson's disease participating in voice and choral singing group therapy versus a music appreciation activity. *2018 International Congress.*

Miller N., Noble E., Jones D., Burn D. (2006). Life with communication changes in Parkinson's disease. *Age and Ageing* 2006;35:235–239.

Moss H., Lynch J., O'Donoghue J. (2017). Exploring the perceived health benefits of singing in a choir: an nternational cross-sectional mixed-methods study. *Sage Journals* doi: doi.org/10.1177/1757913917739652

Naik G.S., Gaur G.S., Pal G.K. (2018). Effect of modified slow breathing exercise on perceived stress and basal cardiovascular parameters. *International Journal of Yoga*. 2018; 11(1): 53–58 doi: 10.4103/ijoy. IJOY_41_16: 10.4103/ijoy.IJOY_41_16

Ong J.C., Manber R., Segal Z., Xia Y., Shapiro S., Wyatt J.K. (2014). A randomized controlled trial of mindfulness meditation for chronic insomnia. *Sleep*. 2014;37(9);1553-63. doi: 10.5665/sleep.4010.

Ozdemir E., Norton A., Schlaug G. (2006). Shared and distinct neural correlates of singing and speaking. *Neurimage*. 2006; 33(2): 628–635

Pacchetti C., Mancini F., Aglieri R., Fundarò C., Martignoni E., and Nappi G. (2000). Active music therapy in Parkinson's disease: an integrative method for motor and emotional rehabilitation. *Psychosomatic Medicine*. 62: 386–393

Pal G., Velkumary S., Madanmohan. (2004). Effect of short-term practice of breathing exercises on autonomic function in normal human volunteers. *Indian J Med Res* 2004;120(2):115–121

Park E., Oh H., Kim T. (2013). The effects of relaxation breathing on procedural pain and anxiety during burn care. *Burns*. 2013; 39(6):1101-1106. doi.org/10.1016/j.burns.2013.01.006

Pearce E., Launay J., Dunbar R.I.M. (2015). The ice-breaker effect: singing mediates fast social bonding. *Royal Society Open Science*. doi: dx.doi. org/10.1098/rsos.150221

Pennington S., Snell K., Lee M., Walker R. (2010). The cause of death in idiopathic Parkinson's disease. *Parkinsonism Relat Disord*. 16(7):434–437

Perciavalle V., Blandini M., Fecarotta P., Buscemi A., Di Corrado D., Bertolo L., Fichera F., Coco M. (2016). The role of deep breathing on stress. *Neurol Sci.* doi: 10.1007s10072-016-2790–2798

Prigatano G.P., Maier F., Burns R.S. (2010). Anosognosia and Parkinson's disease. In: G P Prigatano (ed). *The study of anosognosia.* Oxford: Oxford University Press. pp.159–169

Proud E.L., Morris M.E. (2010). Skilled hand dexterity in Parkinson's disease: Effect of adding a concurrent task. *Arch Phys Med Rehabil* 2010: 91: 794–799

Quinn L., Busse M., Dal Bello-Haas V. (2013). Management of upper extremity disfunction in people with Parkinson disease and Huntington disease: Facilitating outcomes across the disease lifespan. *J Hand Ther* 2013; 26: 148–154

Russo M A., Santarelli D M., O'Rourke D. (2017). The physiological effects of slow breathing in the healthy human. *Breathe* 2017 13:2980309. doi: 10.1183/20734735.009817

Salimpoor V.N., van den Bosch I., Kovacevic N., McIntosh A.R., Dagher A., Zatorre R.J. (2013). Interactions between the nucleus accumbens and auditory cortices predict music reward value. *Science* 340; 2144-2162. doi: 10.1126/science.1231059

Schladt T.M., Nordmann G.C., Emilius R., Kudielka, B.M., de Jong T.R., Neumann I D. (2017). Choir versus solo singing: effects on mood and salivary oxytocin and cortisol concentrations. *Frontiers in Human Neuroscience.* 2017; 11:430.

Shakespeare T., Whieldon A. (2017). Singing your heart out: community singing as part of mental health recovery. *Medical Humanities*, 2017; medhum-2017-011195. doi: 10.1136//medhum-2017-011195

Stegemoller E.L., Radig H., Hibbing P., Wingate J., Sapienza C. (2017). Effects of singing on voice, respiratory control and quality of life in persons with Parkinson's disease. *Disability and Rehabilitation.* 2017; 39(6): 594-600. doi: doi.org/10.3109/09638288.2016.1152610

Tamplin J., Morris M.E., Marigliani C., Baker F.A., Vogel A.P. (2019). ParkinSong: A controlled trial of singing-based therapy for Parkinson's Disease. *Neurorehabilitation and Neurol Repair.* doi: doi. org/10.1177/1545968319847948

Tanner M., Rammage L., Liu Lili. (2016). Does singing and vocal strengthening improve vocal ability in people with Parkinson's disease? *An International Journal for Research, Policy and Practice.* 2016;8(3). doi: doi.org /10.1080/17533015.2015.1088047

Thaut M.H., McIntosh K.W., McIntosh G.C., Hoemburg V. (2001). Auditory rhythmicity enhances movement and speech motor control in patients with Parkinson's disease. *Functional Neurology,* 16,163–172

Thaut M H., Hoemberg V. (Eds) (2014). *Handbook of Neurologic Music therapy.* Oxford University Press.

Tillerson J.L., Cohen A.D., Caudle W.M., Zigmond M.J., Schallert T., Miller G.W. (2002). Forced nonuse in unilateral parkinsonian rats exacerbates injury. *J Neurosci* 2002; 22(15): 6790–6799.

Tomokolnoue Y.H. (2012). The effects of deep breathing on 'tension-anxiety' and fatigue in cancer patients undergoing adjuvant chemotherapy. *Complementary Therapies in Clinical Practice.* 2012:18(2) 94–98. doi. org/10.1016/j.ctcp.2011.10.001

Torsney K.M., Forsyth D. (2017). Respiratory dysfunction in Parkinson's disease. *J R Coll Physicians Edinb.*

Tripoliti E., Zrinzo L., Martinez-Torres I., Frost E., Pinto S., Foltynie T., Holl E., Petersen E., Roughton M., Hariz M.I., Limousin P. (2011). Effects of subthalamic stimulation on speech of consecutive patients with Parkinson's disease. *Neurology*, 76: 80–86.

Tuelings H.L., Contreras-Vidal J.L., Stelmach G.E., Adler C.H. (1997). Parkinsonism reduces coordination of fingers, wrist and arm in fine motor control. *Exp Neurol* 1997; 146: 159–170

Viallet F., Meynadier Y., Lagrue B., Mignard P. (2000). The reductions of tonal range and of average pitch during speech production in "off" parkinsonisms are restored by L-DOPA. *Mov Disord* 2000;15:S131

Vik B.M.D., Skeie G.O., Vikane E., Specht K. (2018). Effects of music production on cortical plasticity within cognitive rehabilitation of patients with mild traumatic brain injury. *Brain Injury*. 32(5): 634–643. doi: 10.1080/02699052.2018.1431842

Wan C.Y., Ruber T., Hoohmann A., Schlaug G. (2010). The therapeutic effects of singing in neurological disorders. *Music Percept.*2010; 27(4): 287–295. doi: 10.1525/mp.2010.27.4.287

Weltzberg E., Lundberg J.O. (2002). Humming greatly increases nasal nitric oxide. *Am J Respit Crit Med* 2002; 166(2): 144–145. doi: 10.1164/rccm.200202-138BC

Wessel J. (2004). The effectiveness of hand exercises for persons with rheumatoid arthritis: A systematic review. *J Hand Ther* 2004; 17: 174–180.

Yorkston K.M., Miller R.M., Strand E.A. (2004). Management of speech and swallowing in degenerative diseases. *Austin, Texas*: pro-e:2004

Zaccaro A., Piarulli A., Laurino M., Garbella E., Menicucci D., Neri B., Gemignani A. (2018). How breath-control can change your life: a systematic review on psycho-physiological correlates of slow breathing. *Frontiers in Human Neuroscience*. doi: 10.3389/fohum.2018.00353

Zatorre R.J., Chen J.L., Penhune V.B. (2007). When the brain plays music: auditor-motor interactions in music perception and production. *Nature Reviews Neuroscience.* 8: 547–558